M000282337

BREAK
YOUR
PRESCRIBED
ADDICTION

A Guide To Coming Off Tranquilizers, Antidepressants (S.S.R.I.s, M.A.O.s) & More With Amino Acids and Nutrient Therapy

**Billie Jay Sahley, Ph.D., and
Katherine M. Birkner, C.R.N.A., Ph.D.**

Pain & Stress Publications®
San Antonio, Texas
2004

Note to Readers

This material is not intended to replace services of a physician, nor is it meant to encourage diagnosis and treatment of illness, disease, or other medical problems by the layman. This book should not be regarded as a substitute for professional medical treatment and while every care is taken to ensure the accuracy of the content, the authors and the publisher cannot accept legal responsibility for any problem arising out of experimentation with the methods described. Any application of the recommendations set forth in the following pages is at the reader's discretion and sole risk. If you are under a physician's care for any condition, he or she can advise you as to whether the programs described in this book are suitable for you.

This publication has been compiled through research resources at The Pain & Stress Center, San Antonio, Texas 78229.

4th Edition
Printed in San Antonio, Texas (U.S.A.)

Additional copies may be ordered from:
The Pain & Stress Center
5282 Medical Drive, Suite 160, San Antonio, Texas
78229-5379
1-800-669-2256
http://www.painstresscenter.com

Library of Congress Catalog Card Number: 2004095361
ISBN: 1-889391-27-1

Dedicated . . .

To a new generation of physicians, therapists, professionals, and educators who seek to find the natural alternative that frees the addicted from the prison of prescription drugs and gives them God's greatest gift—the freedom to make a choice.

To my beloved mother, who started me on the path of understanding the power of the mind and using it.

To a little boy named Scooter.

And to the Lord, for always lighting our paths.

> There is no such thing as an impossible dream.
> If you believe it, you can make it happen.

Acknowledgements

Many professional angels dedicated themselves to making the update of this book possible—countless hours of research, phone calls, and writing needed to bring this book up-to-date with the latest research and information.

One special angel is Jule Freeman, R.M.T., C.N.C. candidate, who lived it daily and many nights until the end. Jule's devoted efforts are on each page to bring forth the information to help those in need of living prescription drug-free.

Linda Volpenhein, Laura Madden, and Mary Randolph spread angel dust in all of their efforts. We thank them all for their dedication and caring.

Our sincere appreciation and thanks to:

The many special friends who support our research including Laurie Allen, D.C., Daniel G. Amen, M.D., Elliott Balbert, Peter Breggin, M.D., Phyllis Bronson, Ph.D., Jay S. Cohen, M.D., Julie Davis, N.C., Martin Feldman, M.D., O.L. Fikes, D.C., John Gosling, M.D., Linda Griffith, R.N., Paul Lynn, M.D., Doris Rapp, M.D., Max Ricketts, Jr, Sherry Rogers, M.D., Dennis Remington, M.D., Barbara Swasey, R.D., Scott J. Smith, Annemarie Welch, M.D., Julian Whitaker, M.D., and the many physicians, R.N.s, chiropractors, and professionals across the country using orthomolecular medicine who share their research and give us constant encouragement.

Our patients who teach us or challenge us everyday.

Contents

Drugs Include:

Charts

Introduction

A basic medical principle is that when people take a chemical affecting the central nervous system, and they take it daily for awhile, dependency may develop or, if the chemical is stopped abruptly, withdrawal symptoms may occur. Look no further than , caffeine, or nicotine—all are characterized by a psychological and often physiological need to continue using these substances, and many people encounter problems when they try to stop. The same problems commonly occur with prescription drugs affecting the nervous system.

Not everyone experiences dependency or withdrawal phenomena. Individual variation is common in how people respond to drugs and which drugs they respond to best. Similarly, there's wide variation in how people respond when trying to discontinue drugs. Some people can smoke for decades and then stop without a hitch. Others try to stop again and again but never can overcome the nagging symptoms of withdrawal. It's not just a question of willpower, but also of chemistry—the chemistry of the individual and the chemistry of the drug.

I was a medical student when Valium became available. It was clearly superior and safer than the barbiturates people were using, but it was addictive, contrary to the advertising claims. After being the #1 drug in America for years, stories of dependency and withdrawal reactions appeared, and people and doctors became concerned. But we should have known from the start that the overuse of Valium would create problems with dependency and

withdrawal. Any substance that alters brain chemistry,
when taken daily, will inevitably cause dependency and
withdrawal problems in some people.

With Valium falling into disfavor, other companies
rushed to capture the big anti-anxiety drug market.
Xanax won based on advertising that emphasized it was
short-acting, as opposed to long-acting Valium. This
short-acting property was supposed to prevent buildup of
Xanax in people's bloodstreams and tissues, and doctors
fell for this line. But anyone familiar with pharmacology
knew that Xanax, because it was short-acting, might pose
greater risks than Valium.

Why? The risk and severity of withdrawal reactions are
influenced by three major factors: how much you've been
taking, how long you've been taking it, and how quickly
the drug leaves your system. The quicker the drug leaves,
the more severe the reaction. With long-acting drugs, the
brain has more time to adjust. Short-acting drugs leave
little time for adjustment; therefore, rebound phenomena
and withdrawal reactions can be more common and more
severe. This is exactly what I saw with Xanax, which
caused more severe withdrawal reactions more often than
I ever saw with Valium. Indeed, as Dr. Sahley suggests,
handling withdrawal reactions with Xanax often requires
the use of a long-acting drug like Valium.

Similar problems are seen with sleep medications.
Halcion (triazolam) works fine for some people, but with
others, it is so short-acting and leaves the system so
abruptly, people awaken at 3 AM and are unable to fall
back to sleep. The same trend has been seen with antidepressants, where the recognition of withdrawal reactions
came slowly, but now is well founded. And it's well known
that short-acting antidepressants like Paxil and Zoloft
are more prone to withdrawal reactions when stopped

abruptly than long-acting Prozac.

Does this mean long-acting drugs are better than short-acting ones? No. In fact, short-acting drugs are often easier to use because they don't quietly build up in the system. That's why, although Prozac was the first of the new serotonin-enhancing antidepressants (SSRIs), short-acting Zoloft and Paxil are preferred by many experts. That's why Halcion and Ambien, short-acting sleep remedies, are preferred over older, long-acting Dalmane, which left many people with a hangover in the morning.

The point is, we're all different, and people respond differently to medications. But no matter which type of medication you use, any regular, long-term use of drugs or other substances affecting the central nervous system can cause dependency or withdrawal reactions in a substantial percentage of people.

How can you avoid dependency? By using the very lowest doses necessary. Believe it or not, the doses your doctor prescribes, which he gets directly from the drug's package insert or *Physicians' Desk Reference* (PDR), may not be the lowest effective doses. As I've written in more than a dozen medical journal articles and in *Over Dose: The Case Against The Drug Companies* (Tarcher/Putnam 2001), drug research and marketing is directed toward the *average* person. This leads to the use of drug doses that are unnecessarily strong for millions of people. For example, the standard starting dose of Prozac is 20 mg/day, but even before Prozac was approved, it was shown 5 mg/day was effective for a significant number of depressed patients. Similarly, in my experience, the standard doses of Xanax are too high, and the guidelines for Xanax to treat panic disorder are downright dangerous.

If dependency and withdrawal are a function of the amount of drug taken, then it's important for you to be sure you are receiving the very lowest dose of any drug or any supplement. Any chemical—drug or supplement—that affects the central nervous system should be used wisely, which means at the lowest amount necessary to accomplish the goal. Some people need low doses and others need higher doses, but what's important is you get the right dose for you.

Should you avoid treatment altogether? I am not anti-drug or anti-treatment. I'm for careful, intelligent, low-risk treatment. I'm for using natural methods when possible, and if they don't suffice, or if your condition is severe and needs immediate, intensive treatment, I'm for using proven-effective prescription drugs. Life is stressful. Chemical imbalances are real. Traumas are part of everyone's life. Major loss and physical illness impact the mind and alter brain chemistry. It is a godsend we have better treatments today. Our drugs are better and safer, even if they aren't without risk, and people like Dr. Sahley are broadening our choices with natural remedies.

Using supplements and medications safely often means simply using common sense. Whenever I discontinued a drug affecting the nervous system, I had patients do so gradually. I didn't need to wait for reports about withdrawal reactions with Valium or Paxil to know that gradual reduction is much safer than stopping abruptly. Doctors and patients shouldn't have to wait a decade for medical science to decide that withdrawal reactions are real after all. Doctors believe—erroneously— that if a side effect isn't listed in a drug's package insert, the drug just can't be causing the problem. Most doctors don't know that many important side effects aren't listed in package inserts, which are based on just a few pre-approval studies. Most doctors don't know that 51% of all drugs are ultimately found to have major side effects that weren't identified in early research. Thus, dependency and withdrawal phenomena shouldn't surprise us with any drug that affects the central nervous system, whether or not a drug manufacturer's package insert or PDR description acknowledges it.

Similarly, we can't always wait for the medical-pharmaceutical system to consider safer, natural remedies. The big money in medical research goes to the development and marketing of patented, profitable, prescription products. The influence of the drug industry is so great, more than 95% of all information that doctors receive about treatments comes from the drug industry, and most of this information is directed toward the use of prescription drugs. Thus, is it any surprise that doctors often treat drug side effects with more drugs? Or that doctors often treat the insomnia from antidepressants with sleep remedies, and they treat the agitation with Xanax. That's what doctors do—even good, caring doctors—because that's what doctors know. This is why it's so important that Dr. Sahley and others are researching natural methods for solving the same problems.

Most people don't like taking medications and, if they must, they want to take as little as possible. Most people prefer natural remedies over prescription drugs. If Valium and Xanax can increase GABA, why not consider GABA itself? If Prozac and Zoloft can increase serotonin, why not consider the amino acids that are the precursors of serotonin? And when withdrawal is a problem, why not use natural methods when possible?

Today, we have two branches of medicine: mainstream and alternative. But you shouldn't have to go to two doctors to get one complete picture. All doctors should be versed in traditional and alternative methods. All doctors should know about natural alternatives that can be used instead of prescription drugs, and when to use them for best results. Medical research should be guided to first identify the safest, most physiologic, natural methods, and then prescription drugs. But that's not how the system works today. So you have to become your own researcher. You have to seek independent sources of good information that make sense medically. And if you find information that makes sense, spread the word and even tell your doctor. The free flow of information is the antidote to the mainstream healthcare system's over-dependence on prescription drugs.

The fact that you are reading this book means you are unsatisfied with the current healthcare system and you want to empower yourself. You aren't alone. Most people are unsatisfied, with good reason. In 2001, Americans filled 3.2 billion prescriptions, 12 for every man, woman, and child in America. Prescription drugs do a lot of good, but they also are overused and cause a lot of unnecessary harm. The movement toward natural remedies can offset this over-reliance on prescription drugs and help bring balance to the system and better methods to individuals. This is an important goal, today more than ever as more and more adults and children are placed on prescription drugs. So if you find the advice in this book helpful, spread the word. If we are to change the system, it will have to begin with us.

Jay S. Cohen, M.D.
Associate Professor (voluntary)
Dept. of Family and Preventive Medicine and of Psychiatry
University of California, San Diego
Author: *Over Dose: The Case Against The Drug Companies*

A Long Journey

Today, drug companies spend millions of dollars publicizing and promoting pharmaceuticals rather than researching them. They want to convince all of us that their products are useful and beneficial so doctors will prescribe them, and we will demand them. This industry flourishes on illness, not on wellness. It has no significant financial incentive to strive for a healthy and drug-free society.

Most medical doctors do not appreciate the extent to which nutrition plays in well-being. Their educational experience concerning nutrition proves to be only superficial. Medical doctors' studies are generally limited to less than one semester of study, learning caloric requirements and recommended dietary allowances to prevent the onset of disease states.

Everyone has problems. Drugs make these problems unmanageable, unresolvable, and unbearable. Drug therapy is very hazardous to one's mental and physical health. Drug users are thirty times more likely to commit suicide than the norm. No one ever fully recovers from anxiety, insomnia, or depression while on drugs whether they take drugs in the form of alcohol, recreational or pharmaceutical drugs.

In the early sixties, to meet the commercial demand for anxiety relief, the pharmaceutical giants began marketing a new class of so-called *minor* tranquilizers/sedatives: the benzodiazepines. The most popular brand names in this class of drugs include Ativan, Dalmane, Halcion, Lexotan,

Librium, Tranxene, Valium, and Xanax. Benzodiazepines exist as commercial products, not because of any demonstrated efficacy in curing anxiety and insomnia. They exist because of the tremendous profits they generate for the people that manufacture, promote, market, and prescribe them. These profits are made possible due to the inherent addictive potential and proprietary patent protection of this merchandise.

My own experience with panic attacks and prescription drug addiction made me a victim of pharmaceutical medicine and a refugee from the mainstream medical establishment, which prescribes the toxic chemical compounds out of ignorance.

My condition was characterized by free-floating anxiety and panic attacks, attacks which came without warning and seemingly without provocation. They simulate heart attacks. Similarly, 30% of U.S. cardiac emergency room admissions actually prove to be panic attacks disguised as heart attacks.

Thanks to the anxiety provoking effect of many pharmaceuticals and sucrose-laden processed foods of the modern supermarket, anxiety disorders are epidemic in the United States and are now considered the number one mental health problem today.

Prescription drug dependents become addicts, in part, because they are unaware of natural alternatives. They base their choices on doctors' prescriptions. These victims go through a very long period of addiction denial because drugs deplete one's will power.

Denial is self-defeating. Addicts, and often their families, deny the addiction. Some never do admit it. To look at the situation honestly would frighten them. Honest, open communication of feelings in a non-judgmental way proves vital to healing.

Public confusion is inevitable. After all, for years we've been led to believe that what a doctor says must be right for us, and anything sold in the pharmacy, especially those drugs made by pharmaceutical companies must be good for us. We, and our doctors, have all come to feel this way, thanks to the one of the world's most effective public relations promotion campaigns led by the pharmaceutical companies.

Sixty-five million tranquilizer prescriptions were written in the United States alone in 1996. As recently as 1995, Americans were consuming 1.5 million pounds of tranquilizers along with 900,000 pounds of barbiturates annually. Unscrupulous practitioners riddle the practices of medicine and psychiatry with a lot of myths, misconceptions and even outright deceptions.

No pill in psychiatric pharmacology that *cures* any psychiatric condition. They all treat symptoms with varying degrees of success, and they all have possible adverse side effects.

The basic requirements of each of your body's many trillion cells, in order to fulfill their quadrillions of functions, are: air, water, and nutrients in very specific and individual amounts. Your body's cells do not require toxic chemical compounds. Drugs operate by blocking metabolic reactions. Nutrients work by *facilitating* metabolic reactions.

The therapeutic approach outlined herein deals with remedying the cause(s) of an altered chemistry, rather than treating the condition symptomatically. The roots of anxiety and panic lie in chemical imbalances within the body and brain.

Health requires achieving a natural state of harmony and equilibrium between the body's systems. When a person reaches this state, an efficient and balanced flow of electro-chemical energy within the nerve and energy pathways creates a stable and unified mind-body system that can effectively deal with life's situations. The mind-body must be viewed as an interrelated whole, with the realization that any action on one part of the mind-body affects all other parts.

You must accept personal responsibility for achieving your own personal state of well-being. If you suffer from anxiety, you must follow a constructive path out of the panic state. The power to live anxiety-and drug-free is within you—you are your own master.

Those persons operating under the influence of pharmaceutical mood-altering drugs, from antihypertensives and antihistamines to tranquilizers and antidepressants, may act and appear cognitive and rational. However, with respect to their medication or treatment, they may exhibit anxiety, depression, confusion, indecisiveness, or obsessiveness and wish to continue clinging to their medication out of fear. If you are one of these people, put a face on your fear, question what you are afraid of and why. You may even intellectually accept that the medication is counter-productive and verbalize wanting to discontinue the drug therapy. However, the vicious, addictive process can disable you from willfully quitting.

Firm, supportive, and communicative confrontation and management is required to help someone back to health. Create a controlled environment under the supervision of a health professional experienced in successfully treating the particular condition(s) of you or your loved one. Orthomolecular therapists and doctors throughout the U.S. specialize in drug withdrawal. And numerous support groups are open to the public.

The term, vitamins, literally means organic compounds essential for life. Without them, we die. Due to metabolic differences, some of us require more nutrients than others. Last year, while no Americans died from vitamin overdose, more Americans died of prescription pharmaceutical side effects than from automobile accidents.

For the millions suffering from prescription drug dependence, orthomolecular therapy offers an alternative that can enhance life and well-being without dependence.

Max Ricketts, Jr.
Author of *The Great Anxiety Escape*

1
What is Addiction?

*Millions have died and millions
will die because of their addiction.*

Addictions affect one out of three people. In the United States alone, more than fifteen million people are affected by the use of some type of toxic substance. It is well established that tranquilizers, antidepressants, pain medication, substance abuse, and alcohol constitute a major health problem in the U.S. Approximately 300,000 men, women, and children will die prematurely every year from a wide range of prescription drug overdoses, abuse of drugs, alcohol, and substance-related problems. Addictions affect people from all social classes, degrees of intelligence, and professional levels.

According to the President's Commission on Mental Health, a quarter of the citizens in the U.S. suffer from some type of severe emotional stress. Another study shows that 80% of all Americans feel the need to reduce stress in their daily lives. *Harrison's Principles of Internal Medicine,* a medical text, states 50 to 80% of all disease is stress induced. All stress-related conditions are similar whether manifested as psychiatric or general medical problems. Does stress lead to addiction? YES!

A cry for help from the American public has gone out: How can they reduce the harmful impact of stress on their physical and mental well-being? Many have come to expect instant relief from stressful emotions and negative feelings. If you swallow one pill or a combination of prescription pills the relief you feel is only brief. When you need psychiatric drugs for quick relief from stressful situations, you risk the possibility of emotional and physical dependence. Records reflect drugs—and a greater inclination to try them, once or twice or perhaps sporadically—fit conveniently into our stress-filled society. These substances allow the manipulation of moods by simply providing a brief escape for the user.

All substances of abuse either elevate or decrease consciousness and often intensify depressed moods. With escape the primary factor, the drug of choice will be the one the user feels will give instant relief. An addicted person

U.S. Top 32 Most Abused Substances (Mood Altering) in 2002

Alcohol-in-combination

Cocaine

Marijuana

Alprazolam (Xanax)

Acetaminophen/ Hydrocodone

Amphetamines

Clonazepam (Klonopin)

Ibuprofen (Motrin)

Oxycodeine (OxyContin, Tylox, Percocet, Percodan)

Methamphetamines

Methadone

Diazepam (Valium)

Lorazepam (Ativan)

Trazodone (Desyrel)

Paroxetine (Paxil)

Zolpidem (Ambien)

Aspirin

Sertraline (Zoloft)

PCP (Angel Dust)

Quetiapine (Seroquel)

Fluoxetine (Prozac)

Venlafaxine (Effexor)

Diphenhydramine (Benadryl)

Carisoprodol (Soma)

Citalopram (Celexa)

Naproxyn (Naproxyn)

Amitriptyline (Elavil)

Olanzapine (Zyprexa)

Acetaminphen/Propoxyphene (Darvocet N, Darvon)

Bupropion (Zyban/ Wellbutrin)

MDMA (Ecstasy)

Risperidone (Risperdal)

Source: Drug Abuse Warning Network Emergency Room Data., 2002.
Tables 2.2.0; 2.4.0;2.6.0;2.7.0; 2.8.0; 2.10.0.

will always satisfy the addiction before he can move on to do anything else.

The newest antidepressant drugs known as Selective Serotonin Reuptake Inhibitors (SSRIs) pose a new and different addiction problem. Although these drugs are not habit-forming in the ways of tranquilizers and pain medications, once started, severe withdrawal symptoms force people to continue taking these drugs long past their usefulness.

Everyone experiences challenges and problems in their lives. Antidepressants, tranquilizers, pain pills, drugs, and alcohol make you feel these problems are not pressing. You can put your worries and your life on hold. In reality prescription drugs and alcohol make problems unmanageable, irresolvable, and unbearable. Psychiatric drug and street drug users are thirty times more likely to commit suicide than the norm.

Using mind-altering drugs ranks as one of the most hazardous activities in the world today. There is no such thing as a safe prescription medication. According to Thomas J. Moore in his best seller, *Prescription for Disaster,* "More than a million prescriptions are written every hour of the working day; in a year's time eight prescriptions have been written for *every man, woman, and child in the United States.*" All research statistics demonstrate there is a major problem in this country with prescription medication abuse.

What predisposes a person to choose a particular substance? The drugs availability through prescriptions or contacts, and finding the funds to pay for it. This is especially evident among teens and those even younger. We live in an addictive society, a society that has all the characteristics and exhibits all the effects of prescribed addiction.

The pervasive use of psychiatric drugs has reached an all time high in the U.S. Last year Xanax (Alprazolam) was right at the top of the more than 80 million prescriptions for benzodiazepines that were handed to unsuspecting consumers. The primary cause of the addiction problem is not the psychological illness, but physical addiction. The body and brain anticipate the feelings of dullness, no fear or anxiety, just passive existence.

Those with an addiction problem become unaware of what is going on around them. They don't have to deal with anger, pain, depression, grief, love, or joy. The drugs cover-up feelings so the addict does not have to think or feel. The addicted person stops relying on his knowledge and sense and relies on confused perceptions. Those with fear, panic, and anxiety live from one pill to the next. Their only goal is to quiet the panic. As addiction and dependence take over many lose contact with others around them, withdrawing into their own world of antidepressants, tranquilizers, and pain pills.

Abuse of and dependence on benzodiazepines such as Xanax, Klonopin, Valium, or Buspar can occur alone or in conjunction with the use of other drugs. Benzodiazepines used either alone or in combination with other prescriptions or alcohol may result in the loss of coordination, concentration, and memory. Users can display mood swings, especially angry outbursts. Many times these angry outbursts are accompanied by fear of not having the next dose.

Addictive substances dull and distort sensory input and output. The user neither receives information clearly nor processes it correctly. Since chemically dependent people are not in touch with themselves, they present a distorted self to the world. Addicts con people and eventually lose the ability to become intimate with others, even those they are closest to and love most—their family and friends.

Chemical dependent people know something is very wrong, but their distorted thinking tells them that it could not possibly be their fault. This kind of thinking also tells them that they cannot make things right—that someone else will have to do it for them. An addiction absolves the user from having to take responsibility for their lives, and permits the assumption that someone or something outside themselves will swoop down to make things better or help them deal with their problems. Since addicts tend to be dependent and feel increasingly powerless and bad about themselves, the notion that they can take responsibility for their lives is inconceivable to them.

The longer the addict waits to be rescued, the worse the dependency becomes. Regardless of what they are addicted to, it takes more and more to create the desired effect. Before recovery can take place, the individual must often hit bottom. At this time a new sense of reality surfaces, they no longer want to hide their addiction; they want help.

The prescription addict finds it staggering to come to terms with the possibility that he could be addicted to more than one drug, and therefore must recover from multiple drugs. The addicted person cannot remain static; he must either get better or worse. Both addiction and recovery processes require time and help.

The addicted personality has been enslaved—a prisoner of his own mind, condemned by his own guilt, fear, and fear of failure. This is one of the reasons he must hit bottom before admitting he is out of control and needs help with his fears—fear of living, fear of loss of control. Once in the process of recovery, the addict must not concern himself with how he got there. He must focus on recovery, living one day at a time. He cannot allow fear of the future to set in, as this leads to almost certain failure. Those with an addiction history grieve for the past and all the time they wasted. Until their brain chemistry is restored, they live in fear of panic, anxiety, depression, and pain. Fear of the future brings forth a new set of problems, anxieties, fears, and phobias. Now he must become responsible and face the realities he has avoided, denied, and pushed aside.

The most important and enduring part of the global response to the addiction problem has been intellectual. Substance abuse therapists and researchers around the world have sought to understand why people try to escape through the use of drugs and alcohol.

Researchers found a specific receptor in the brain for morphine, and they discovered *natural brain chemicals* that fit these receptors. This finding opened the door to a new understanding of the psychiatric profile of substance abusers and their brain function.

Researchers also determined there is a neurochemical imbalance that makes the alcoholic incapable of drinking normally. His body simply does not process alcohol correctly. And unlike other psychoactive drugs, alcohol does not target specific parts of nerve cells or neurons. Instead it seems to enter cell membranes and sabotage the nervous system indiscriminately.

The National Institute of Mental Health (NIMH) is studying how alcohol affects certain cells in the brain to induce a sedative effect. The complex workings of the brain provide a map with unique pathways for the addicted. Although some become sedated, others become agitated, angry, depressed, melancholy, anxious, excited and fearful. The brain chemistry holds the key. Deficiencies or imbalances are thought to be the result of genetic anomalies, metabolic disturbances due to stress, or the destructive effects of prescription drugs, alcohol, or drug abuse.

One theory on addiction, according to Janice Phelps, M.D., is that certain individuals are born with a biochemical defect that predisposes them to addiction. The physiologic flaw begins at least in part in the adrenal glands. This defect consists of a sugar imbalance or dysmetabolism and a chronic biochemical depression or genetic depression. Genetic depression, a chronic physiological and biochemical depression passed from generation to generation in some families, does not necessarily affect all family members. Genetic depression very closely relates to addictiveness, conceivably arising from the same physiological defect in the brain.

Genetic depression may arise in infancy or childhood, or it may not appear until the teen years or even adulthood. It may go unrecognized if it has been present so long that it seems normal for that person; usually the person living with it has become an expert at concealing it.

The signs of genetic depression are many and varied. Signs of this imbalance in infants are seen as indigestion, stomachaches, and craving sweets. In older children, it might be manifested as anxiety, learning disabilities, attention problems, or hyperactivity. In the adult, headaches, backaches, and stomachaches are common, as are anxiety and worry. Sleep disorders, appetite changes, lack of energy, and constant fatigue may also be present. Even changes in sexual response may be related to depression. A defect in the chemical communication from the brain to the adrenals seems to provide the single key to this imbalance.

The signs and symptoms of depression must be recognized, but anxiety and depression are so similar at times that even physicians cannot tell the difference. The relationship between the pituitary-adrenal axis and depression must be understood. Some of the major symptoms include physical pain and symptoms, perhaps even mental illness in the genetically depressed person. With the underlying addictiveness or family history of addiction, many symptoms may be attributed to depression. Many addicted people do not realize they are depressed and have been depressed most of their lives.

According to Dr. Phelps, a good working definition of addiction is as follows, "An addiction is the compulsive and out-of-control use of any chemical substance that can produce recognizable and identifiable unpleasant withdrawal symptoms when use of the substance is stopped. Such addiction is driven by an inborn physiological hunger in the addictive person, and is frequently intimately related to depression." All addicting substances, from sugar to nicotine to narcotics, seem to give short-term relief from depression in the beginning. Later, the same substance aggravates it. The author believes the degree of *normalcy, relaxation* or feeling of well-being a person experiences from an addicting substance probably is related to the individual's degree of depression. There is no doubt that a link exists between depression and addiction. It plays an important role in the overall pattern of addiction and addictive behavior.

No one ever fully recovers from anxiety, insomnia, or depression while on drugs, whether the drugs are in the form of alcohol, street, or pharmaceutical-grade drugs. Stop the drugs, and the anxiety comes back.

Today millions of children are the targets of the pharmaceutical giants and their magic pills. According to a story in *U.S. News and World Report,* August 18, 1998 by Arianna Huffington, "At least 580,000 children are being prescribed antidepressants—and those numbers are likely to increase dramatically." Eli Lilly is on the market with a peppermint flavored Prozac, approved by the FDA for use in children, but many children are being prescribed antidepressants "off label" that have not shown safety or efficacy in children. Huffington's story describes the future treatment of children in America—if they even have the slightest problem or down day.

When does addiction begin? When you're taking a substance that can produce withdrawal symptoms and you have a physical dependency. Ritalin, a powerful stimulant drug, is being passed out at a very early age. Children take Ritalin to calm down, then antidepressants and tranquilizers as teens to perk up. None of these medications do anything to relieve the underlying nutritional deficiencies. By the time they reach twenty they are predisposed to addiction from past use. Everyone has down days, even kids. This is part of normal behavior. Children do not need addictive drugs. They need neurotransmitters to nourish it. The brain is the busiest, yet the most undernourished organ in the body. Drugs do not nourish the brain. They have no nourishment value. Drugs suppress symptoms. Drugs certainly do not nourish.

A story in the *New York Times* August 8, 1997 reported that nearly 600,000 children and adolescents were prescribed Prozac, Paxil, or Zoloft. According to IMS American Ltd., a research organization, Prozac prescriptions for those 13 to 18 years old increased 46% in 1996. Eli Lilly, the Prozac king, reported sales totaled $1.73 billion in the U.S. alone.

Since the adult market for prescribed addiction has become saturated, the drug companies are looking for new markets. Their thrust is aimed directly at our children! Insurance companies will pay for drugs even though not enough is known about how antidepressants work on the growing brain. But they won't pay for amino acids or supplements even when a physician prescribes them, yet the growing brain is desperately in need of nutrients.

Let kids be kids and go through the normal growing pains, experience ups and downs; moreover they learn to verbalize their feelings and resolve problems. Don't drug your children or yourself. Prescription drug dependents become addicted and lost, in large part, because they are unaware of the natural alternatives and orthomolecular therapy. They have been told the only way to stop anxiety, panic, depression, or grief is to take drugs.

Our entire generation has come to believe that any kind of suffering is bad. Millions of Americans believe we should not suffer any type of discomfort, including pain. So, rather than find answers through education and information, they reach for the easy way out and take a pill. By taking a pill it allows them to ignore the problem, escape reality, and never really come to grips with why they suffer and how to resolve it. Prescription addicts live in denial, but denial is self-defeating. Addicts, and often their families as well, deny their dependency.

The late Carl C. Pfeiffer, M.D., Ph.D., renowned for his work in the field of orthomolecular medicine, summed up the challenge in what he calls "Pfeiffer's Law", which states, "We have found that if a drug can be found to do the job of medical healing, a nutrient can be found to do the same job. When we understand how a drug works, we can imitate its action with one of the nutrients."

While unaware of natural alternatives and orthomolecular therapy, prescription drug dependents become addicted because they make choices based on the convention that has taught them to trust their doctor and his medicines. These victims go through a long period of prescribed addiction denial. But denial is self-defeating. Addicts, and often their families as well, deny the addiction.

There appears to be agreement about the presence of the three major elements in the drug abuse problem: the drugs, the people who use them, and the social forces shaping, and in turn being influenced by, all of these. A recently coined term that fits the study of all three of these elements is *social pharmacology*; it now awaits new definitions and delineations of its role in the psychotropic (i.e., mind-altering) drug abuse field.

A new attitude characterizes the thinking of the American public. Even drugs prescribed by a physician may not be good for you, and serious side effects as well as long-term addiction can occur. Those with emotional problems and chronic pain are potential victims of a helpless, hopeless dependency.

· The Council on Patient Information and Education states, "Up to half of all prescription drugs are taken incorrectly." People do not understand how toxic chemicals affect their brain and the pervasiveness of dependency. The abuse of prescription drugs prevails among the most widespread problems in the United States today. People take more than they need because of fear. Fear of anxiety, fear of depression, fear of loneliness, or fear their pain will come back.

When patients are prescribed drugs such as antidepressants, tranquilizers or painkillers physicians typically do not tell them the drug has a potential for dependency much less spend any time counseling the patient concerning the risks for such.

Senior citizens are major targets for prescription drug dependency, especially when they have no family or a reliable source of information. Anxiety, depression, and pain are the three major reasons why they begin taking addictive medications. Most often their first prescription is for a benzodiazepine, the most commonly prescribed medication in the world. When this drug doesn't solve the problem, or in order to relieve the symptoms of side-effects, another drug is prescribed starting the snowball effect of medications leading to more and more medications. Over-

Important Warning: R_X Medications Are Drugs

No drugs in pharmacology cure anxiety, panic, phobias, insomnia, depression, allergies, arthritis, asthma, cardiac, diabetes, hypertension, hyperactivity, or inflammatory conditions, chronic pain, or disease.

Many drugs treat the symptoms of these disorders. However, many prescription drugs have a significant potential for long-term adverse or permanent drug side effects.

When the word *addict* is used, it does not mean just the addict on street drugs. Addict applies to people from all walks of life, all ages, and whole families, who depend on mind-altering drugs to get through life. Even children are not immune if their parents allow them to take prescribed drugs such as antidepressants, tranquilizers, or stimulants; this, in fact, sets up a pattern for a lifetime with a chemical straightjacket.

medication is a major problem for the elderly.

Many seniors come to our office and express concern over the multiple medications they are given. They see not only their primary doctor, but specialists as well. Each doctor gives them multiple prescriptions, but not reporting it to the other. The latest information documents more than 9 million adverse drug reactions and as many as 245,000 hospitalizations. This does not need to happen if physicians would communicate prescription information to each other as well as notify a patient's family members precautions that should be taken.

After the age of 65, a senior metabolizes drugs differently, and this puts them in a high-risk group for a drug reaction. The number one risk factors are sedatives, sleeping pills, and benzodiazepines. When these drugs do not wear off by morning, many seniors are left with a feeling of confusion, memory loss, depression, and an inability to concentrate or focus. In some cases, this results in a fall and the chance of a hip fracture or other broken bones.

In 80% of patients, psychiatric (psychotropic) drugs are never needed. Correcting brain deficiencies resolves the problem. The diet of many seniors today is totally inadequate, and they do not realize they are running on empty and need neurotransmitters. They feel anxious, depressed, or unwanted. Many turn to alcohol. Alcohol, in combination with drugs, makes seniors more vulnerable and end up in a hospital with a drug reaction. To prevent this problem, their doctors and drug companies must do more education. The drug companies spend millions advertising to convince us their drug is the answer, but rarely spend time to educate and inform the consumer about risks, side effects, etc.

Patients often ask about a chemical imbalance. You cannot correct this with a drug. You must put back in the brain what belongs there—neurotransmitters. If your parents or grandparents are taking SSRIs, antidepressants, pain relievers, or muscle relaxants, etc., be aware of the risks and potential problems. Try to explain to them how this negatively affects their brain. Remember, whatever the brain tells the body to do, the body will do!

2
Withdrawal and Recovery

When you want to withdraw from an addictive substance you will probably experience many anxiety-related symptoms. You feel the increasing uncertainty about whether or not you will succeed. Withdrawal reactions vary a great deal from person to person. Some people can reduce the quantity and even drop tranquilizers without any problems. Others experience minor problems, but some have major withdrawal situations. **Use extreme caution when starting *any* drug withdrawal program. Do not begin withdrawal unless you follow a program that advises you how and what to do and what to expect.**

Withdrawal And Recovery Take Time

Addiction does not happen overnight and your system cannot release all the accumulated toxins at once. Only a few drugs give proper therapeutic action. People who regularly take tranquilizers, antidepressants, and pain medication often experience the following side effects: depression, anxiety, headaches, loss of appetite, phobias, stiffness and soreness, sinus pain, confusion, diarrhea or constipation, dizziness, loss of reality, blurred vision, emotional outbursts, anger and rage, slurred speech, lack of coordination, muscle spasms, memory impairment, personality changes, sore or achy joints, and emotional exhaustion.

Withdrawal symptoms can range in severity and intensity from mild anxiety, irritability, and craving for the addicting substances to blackouts and seizures, although the latter are rare. Successfully coping with withdrawal and breaking your addiction depends on:

1. *General health and age.* Younger people commonly have "newer" habits. In addition, they are more resilient and generally have more physical resources to draw on.

2. *Psychological stress load and mental state.* Prerequisites for any successful withdrawal are a positive attitude and freedom from tension.

3. *Length of time of addiction.* Generally, the shorter the addiction, the easier it is to break.

4. *Nature of the substance* to which an individual is addicted.

5. *Dosage or concentration* of the addicted substance or medication, the spacing of dosages and route of administration.

6. *Availability and extent of medical care,* support groups, and family assistance, if needed, that can be expected.

7. *Whether the addiction is part of a peer group milieu.* Often these "friends" can contribute to the problem by peer pressure and your need to fit in.

8. *Personal habits,* including the use of other drugs, medications, or alcohol. In order to have an effective recovery, the amount of toxic chemicals in the body must be reduced.

Recovery Time

The supreme hurdle most people face when detoxing from habit-forming substances is not giving up and feeling helpless and hopeless. *Do not become impatient.* It takes the body time to release all of the chemicals, toxins, and poisons and return to a normal homeostasis.

During use, the benzodiazepines and tranquilizers take the biggest toll on your brain and body. They cause physical and psychological dependence—more so than do alcohol, cocaine, or heroin.

The number one question for those going into recovery is, "How long will it take before I am free?" Each person is biochemically unique, so the answer depends on your own biological makeup and the condition of your immune system. For some, recovery could take only weeks, others months, but with some it could be a year or more before all of the adverse symptoms are completely gone. Symptoms in the later months will not be as severe as in the beginning, but there are some nagging effects that can linger.

At first, coping with stressful situations may not be easy after withdrawal has begun. Stress and anxiety during withdrawal will be eased by the use of amino acids such as GABA, L–T (L-Theanine complex), 5-HTP, Super BNC, tyrosine, glutamine, lysine, methionine, Vitamin B6 (pyridoxine), and magnesium. The immune system must be restored and constant positive reinforcement given by a therapist, friends, and family.

Freedom From Pills

After taking tranquilizers, pain pills, or antidepressants

Sample Dose Reduction

Starting Total Dose is 8 mg			
Week 1	6 mg	Week 5	0.5 mg
Week 2	4 mg	Week 6	0.25 mg
Week 3	2 mg	Week 7	OFF
Week 4	1 mg		

NEVER Reduce Your Dosage by More than
one-quarter (¼) of the total mg dosage per week!

for a long period, you can experience some or all of the following symptoms:

1. Increased anxiety attacks
2. Panic attacks
3. Depression
4. Personality changes
5. Skin and hair problems
6. Glazed eyes
7. Memory problems
8. Digestive upsets
9. Headaches
10. Constant pain
11. Sleep disorders
12. Weight loss or gain
13. Slow reaction time
14. No interest in sex
15. Dry mouth
16. Palpitations
17. Tremors
18. Constipation
19. Blurred vision
20. Tachycardia
21. Tardive dyskinesia
22. Muscle spasms
23. Irritable Bowel Syndrome
24. Vertigo
25. Mood swings

When you have a chemical dependency, you cannot just stop. You must follow a regular reduction plan along with a complete amino acid and nutrient therapy program, as well as a counseling program. A planned treatment program protects the body and brain from feeling severe symptoms, such as sudden changes in the level of the drug in the bloodstream.

The chronic abuse of psychoactive drugs usually leads to what has been termed *psychological or psychic dependence.* Your attitude and the intensity of your habit, how often you need and use a particular substance are all aspects that need analysis to aid in your recovery. If you have chronic abuse syndrome, you not only have psychological dependence, but also an obsession that affects your emotional makeup, mind, and life-style.

Guilt should never influence recovery; if you have had an anxiety or depression problem and were given these medications by a physician, you were following what you thought was a therapeutic dose. *However, when a drug has been taken continuously for more than 4 to 6 months, it has little therapeutic effect on the original symptoms.* You may only be avoiding withdrawal symptoms by continuing the medication as well as the toxic effects of the drug.

Just as guilt can be a significant factor, so is fear. The withdrawing person needs constant reinforcement so fear does not impede recovery. Behavior therapists are of great assistance in substance abuse recovery. Their constant reassurance helps insure your rehabilitation. Weekly sessions are helpful, if possible. Consult a physician or health care professional regarding a detox program; if the professional anticipates or sees a problem follow the specific instructions carefully. Provide careful attention to complete withdrawal of such drugs in an elderly dependent person. In this situation it should be done only under the supervision of a physician or qualified health care professional.

The speed at which withdrawal is accomplished from any substance depends on what is happening in your life. If you operate machinery, drive, have small children, a stressful job or a sick person dependent on you, then withdraw even more slowly.

Reduction Procedures

Some doctors may recommend hospitalization for withdrawal following a planned program, but many people achieve withdrawal very well at home. If a physician agrees reduction should take place, but fails to recommend a detox schedule, the drug detoxification handbooks used in most psychiatric hospitals recommend a dose reduction of *one-fourth (¹/₄) the daily dose per 7 days.* (Never compare the number of milligrams; 1 mg of one drug cannot be substituted for 1 mg of another drug. For example, 5 mg of

Valium does not equal 5 mg of Halcion or 5 mg of Ativan.)

The body and brain cry and scream wildly at the anticipation of a reduction or not receiving the drugs or substance they are accustomed to receiving. Considering what drugs are suppose to do—for example, relax muscles, control anxiety, or aid sleep—it is understandable that the body and mind object after they have become accustomed to having it present. The rebound reaction, i.e., the opposite of the desired effect, occurs in many people, at least for the period of withdrawal. In the following list of withdrawal symptoms, note that some people may only experience a few of them, especially if they withdraw slowly and use nutrient replacement therapy.

Withdrawal Symptoms
By Addictive Substance

Medications: Weight loss, chills, hiccups, low back pain, muscle twitching, muscle weakness, tremors, weakness, apathy, craving for the medication/substance, delirium, depression, dizziness, fatigue, insomnia, irritability, loss of appetite, nightmares, panic, anger, rage, crawling sensations on skin, seizures, gooseflesh, rashes, incontinence, stomachaches, intestinal cramps, nausea and vomiting, diarrhea, constipation, yawning, bad taste in mouth, aching in ears, runny nose, smelling of unpleasant odors, watery eyes, uncontrolled blinking, rapid movement of the eyes, dilated pupils, double vision, headaches, muscle contraction headaches, increased anxiety, panic or anxiety attacks, agoraphobia, flu-like symptoms, hyperactivity, hallucinations, confusion, sweating, palpitations, slow or rapid pulse, tight chest, abdominal pain, restlessness, increased sensitivity to noise, light, touch, or smell, change in sex interest, impotence, pains in the shoulder, neck, jaw, or face, jitteriness, and shaking.

Caffeine: Irritability, muscle contraction headaches, migraine headaches, runny nose, tinnitus (ringing in the ears), rapid pulse, diarrhea, flushing, stomachaches, cramps, urinary frequency, flushing, apathy, craving for coffee, delirium, depression, drowsiness, inability to concentrate, tension, unsteady gait, chills, fever and sweating, tremors, weakness.

Nicotine: Weight gain, muscle aches, craving for cigarettes/nicotine, delirium, depression, drowsiness, irritability, insomnia, diarrhea, sore gums or tongue, constipation, stomachaches, intestinal cramping, muscle contraction headaches.

Sugar: Anxiety, craving for sugar, delirium, rage, depression, dizziness, hyperactivity, inability to concentrate, irritability, anger, tremors, weakness, muscle contraction headaches, blurred vision, rapid heartbeat.

Barbiturates: Anxiety, sleep disturbances, irritability, restlessness, postural hypotension, delirium, major motor seizures, fever.

All withdrawal symptoms pass in time. Knowledge and acceptance of the withdrawal symptoms can shorten the recovery time. The goal of physical and mental well-being represents a state that an addicted person may not have experienced for many years.

Anxiety

The majority of withdrawal symptoms are demonstrated in the form of anxiety. This is more severe than worrying about the weather. Disabling physical and emotional symptoms prevent the sufferer from leading a normal life. Studies verified that anxiety levels after drugs have been stopped could be six times greater than pre-withdrawal levels; this is known as rebound anxiety.

Tranquilizers make those who are taking them feel as though the part of the brain that deals with anxiety has stopped functioning properly. But the brain does function at an accelerated rate day and night. The feeling of acceleration is a temporary sensation, and with time and recovery, it passes.

Drugs act by stimulating or depressing the normal physiological function of specific organs. Stimulation is an increase in the rate of functional activity of a cell or in the amount of secretion from a gland. Depression denotes a reduction in such activity. Amphetamines and caffeine stimulate the central nervous system (CNS), whereas alcohol and phenobarbital depress the CNS.

Drugs cannot endow a tissue or cell with properties they do not inherently possess. Thus, no drug is capable of stimulating the epithelial cells located in the mouth to release insulin. A drug cannot transform a muscle fiber in such a manner that it functions as a nerve cell. Drugs can only stimulate or depress the normal activity of a nerve or muscle cell. In addition, stimulants such as amphetamines possess a biphasic activity...that is, in moderate doses amphetamines cause *stimulation*, but at higher doses they cause depression. Drugs are unable to restore diseased organs or tissue functions to normal by a direct action.

Your body requires some time for the normal chemical neurotransmitters to be produced and replenished. *Neurotransmitters* are the chemical language of the brain. For normal functioning during withdrawal the brain must produce these neurotransmitters and endorphins. It takes time for the brain's receptor sites to be restored to their normal level especially after extended prescription drug use. Knowledge is power: you need to understand these processes and know that the capability is there to control anxious messages, stress, and depression, and give the brain time to recover.

Withdrawal Reactions

Many withdrawal symptoms are due to rebound anxiety according to the *Oxford Textbook of Psychiatry*. Anxiety neuroses have both physical and psychological symptoms. The psychological symptoms include fearful anticipation, irritability, difficulty in concentrating, sensitivity to noise, and a feeling of restlessness. People often complain of poor memory, probably due to lack of concentration.

Repetitious thoughts make up an important part of anxiety neuroses. These are often provoked by awareness of the autonomic over-activity; for example, a patient feels his heart beating fast or pounding in his chest and fears a heart attack. Thoughts of this nature will probably prolong the condition.

The appearance of someone with anxiety neurosis is distinctive. His face appears strained, with a furrowed brow; he is restless and frequently shaky; his posture is tense, his skin looks pale, and often he will sweat from his hands, feet, and armpits. There is also increased tension in the skeletal muscles or overstimulation of the sympathetic nervous system. The list of symptoms is extensive and is grouped according to systems in the body.

Symptoms related to the *gastrointestinal system* include rumbling of intestinal gases, frequent or loose bowel movements, excessive air swallowing, epigastric pain (under sternum or breastbone), dry mouth, and feelings of *butterflies* in the stomach.

Cardiovascular symptoms include palpitations, an awareness of missed or irregular heartbeats, throbbing in the neck, feeling of discomfort or pain over the heart or chest, increased or rapid pulse.

Common *respiratory* symptoms include hyperventilation, a feeling of constriction in the chest, and difficulty in catching the breath.

Genitourinary symptoms are increased frequency and urgency of urination, failure of erection, and lack of sexual interest. Women may complain of increased menstrual discomfort or difficulty, and sometimes absence of menstruation.

Other complaints related to the functions of the central nervous system including depression, ringing in the ears, dizziness, headaches, prickling sensations, blurred vision, muscular tension in back and shoulders; muscle pain, sleep disturbances such as insomnia, then intermittent awakening, and unpleasant dreams; depersonalization, not feeling in touch with reality, lack of concentration, hyperactivity, memory loss, rage, panic attacks, noise sensitivity, and unsteady gait. Some people develop pins and needles in their extremities, electricity shooting through their bodies, or shaky legs that last for months to years after withdrawing from the drug.

Medication Withdrawal Procedure

Learn all that you can about any drug you are taking. Check with your pharmacist, physician, *Physicians' Desk Reference* or other reference books on the medication or drug. ***Ask questions. DO NOT be intimidated.***

You can begin by gathering the following information:

1. Determine how addictive the drug is.
2. Determine if *YOU* are addicted. You are if:
   a) Missing even one dosage makes you feel sick, nervous, sad, or you experience a craving for the drug.
   b) You need the drug to function normally.
   c) You begin to require a larger dosage to obtain the same effect.
   d) You continue to use the drug in spite of side effects or other negative reactions.
   e) There is a family history of alcohol or substance abuse.
3. Observe in yourself the withdrawal effects for rapid and slow withdrawal.
4. How long do the withdrawal symptoms last?
5. Can these withdrawal symptoms be minimized without using other medications?

Never stop using a prescription medication unless you have strong feelings and reasons to believe it is harmful to you. Some physicians may not understand your reason for stopping the medication and may feel that you are trying to be an uncooperative patient. They might not support your need to stop and will reassure you that the drug is safe for you for whatever duration you want to take it. But remember that it is *your* body, and the prescription may not always be in your best interest. Don't hesitate to get a second or third opinion from doctors of different orientations and then make your decision based on this information. Drug therapy is a valid medical procedure, but for the most part it is a temporary measure, and to be used only when there is no alternative.

If you decide to quit the drug, know what the withdrawal symptoms are *before* withdrawing. Determine your method and schedule of withdrawal with a physician or qualified health care professional if possible. If your dependency is minor, it probably can be done at home. If your dependency is major, you may need to be in a medical facility for close medical supervision. Be aware that many facilities and physicians use other drugs to withdraw from different substances. *The worst possible treatment is substituting one drug or chemical for another.*

Once you have overcome withdrawal effects, the next step is to remain off the offending drug or substance. Explore amino acid therapy, and add biofeedback, meditation, homeopathic formulas, phenolics (the neutralization of toxic reactions), herbology, deep tissue massage, and acupuncture to remain free of the substance.

Form new habits and friends by joining a support group; these are great support systems and all of the members have had a problem at one time or another. Start exercising (such as walking) everyday to reduce your stress and elevate your endorphins. *Take one day at a time. Keep alert.*

Become an informed educated consumer. Know what you are putting into your body. Ask questions. Do not take any medication unless you know why it is being given to you and what it will do in your body and mind. Always ask what the short-and-long-term side effects are, and chance of addiction. Most drugs have a long list of potential side effects; decide if the benefits out weigh the risks.

3
Benzodiazepines

Benzodiazepines are *highly addictive drugs* with a long list of side effects. The first thing you should know is benzodiazepines *DO NOT* cure anxiety, depression, stress, or insomnia. Benzodiazepines are among the most commonly prescribed medications in the world. They are classified as minor tranquilizers and sedative hypnotics, and prescribed mainly for anxiety, insomnia, muscle relaxant, anticonvulsant, and chronic pain. Despite all of the research and information regarding benzodiazepines, the public does not understand that drugs produce pharmacological tolerance and dependence in a very short time period (in as few as 5 to 6 days); *meaning, you become quickly addicted.*

Clinical research has documented the most effective uses of benzodiazepines are short-term. Beyond two months the effectiveness declines because of the development of dependence, abuse, and tolerance. Doctors continually prescribe benzodiazepines for long periods despite the knowledge of their inherent potential for addiction. Chronic pain patients, because of the nature of their problems, tend to overuse Valium. Doctors prescribe Valium as a muscle relaxant along with other drugs. Long-term drug use sets up the potential for addiction.

According to the *Wall Street Journal*, March 2002, pharmaceutical companies in 2001 spent 2.49 billion dollars advertising to consumers. The resulting profits are made possible by the inherent addictive potential of benzodiazepines and the patent protection of the drug manufacturers who hold the exclusive rights to their formula for seventeen years. Thus, when users become dependent on particular drugs, the pharmaceutical companies make huge profits.

Consumer Reports, January 1993, published an in-depth research report on Xanax, Halcion, and Prozac, the conclusion: ***These drugs do not work!*** Xanax, Halcion and Prozac all have histories of extensive potential for hazardous side effects, including death. In the year 2000, 80 million plus prescriptions for benzodiazepines were filled.

Commonly Prescribed Benzodiazepines

Alprazolam (Xanax)
Chlordiazepoxide (Librium)
Clonazepam (Klonopin)
Diazepam (Valium)
Estazolam (ProSom)
Flunitrazepam (Rohypnol)
Flurazepam (Dalmane)
Halazepam (Paxipam)
Lorazepam (Ativan)
Clorazepate (Tranxene)
Nitrazepam (Mogadon)
Oxazepam (Serax)
Quaqepam (Doral)
Triazolam (Halcion)
Temazepam (Restoril)

Doctors almost always fail to tell patients of the addictive nature of benzodiazepines because they believe controlling the prescription can prevent abuse. The *Physicians' Desk Reference* clearly states even after relatively short-term use (12 weeks), at the doses recommended for the treatment of transient anxiety and anxiety disorder; there is risk of dependence, especially in doses over 4 mgs a day. They go on to say, "Certain adverse clinical events, some life threatening, are a direct consequence to physical dependence to Xanax." Some physicians complicate withdrawal by prescribing other *replacement* drugs. These replacement drugs often impair the withdrawal process.

Are You Hooked?

If three or more of the following characteristics are present over 12 months, a person is considered *dependent* on a substance:

- Tolerance, needing increased doses.
- Withdrawal, becoming physically ill when not using the substance.
- Extension, taking the substance over a longer period of time than intended.
- Failing in efforts to cut down, even knowing use is causing physical or psychological trouble.
- Spending excessive time getting the substance or recovering from its effects.
- Giving up professional or social activities because of substance use.

Source: *American Psychiatric Association's Diagnostic and Statistical Manual of Mental Disorders*

After a few weeks of regular use, benzodiazepines become the *cause* of anxiety, insomnia, panic and fear as a result of tolerance. Tolerance occurs as the body responds to the continued presence of a drug by a series of adjustments. In the case of benzodiazepines the body adjusts to the drug by decreasing GABA receptors in an attempt to restore the balance between excitatory and inhibitory neurotransmitters. Neurotransmitters in the brain do not function independently; they work in harmony with each other and when you artificially raise or lower one, other neurotransmitter levels will be affected. When tolerance develops withdrawal symptoms appear even though continuing to take the drug. The major symptom of withdrawal from benzodiazepines is anxiety, followed by insomnia, which are the two most common reasons these drugs are prescribed in the first place. When patients return to their doctor with complaints of recurring anxiety he will most often increase the dose of benzodiazepine or add an additional medication to take.

There are a large number of benzodiazepines available, differing in potency and speed of elimination. Speed of elimination is described as a drug's *half-life*, which is the amount of time it takes the body to eliminate half of the drug. Alprazolam (Xanax) has a half-life of six to 12

Adverse Effects of Benzodiazepine Use

- Drowsiness, poor concentration, lack of coordination, muscle weakness, and mental confusion.
- Potential for dangerous drug interactions.
- Impairs memory in the ability to learn new information as well as remembering recent events.
- Can have stimulant effect in some individuals causing rage and violent behavior.
- Depression and the inability to feel pleasure or pain.
- Addiction can develop in as little as a few weeks of repeated use.
- Tolerance to the drug develops quickly, requiring higher doses or the addition of more drugs.

hours, while Diazepam's (Valium) half-life is 20 to 100 hours. This means half of the active ingredients in a single dose of Diazepam are still in your system up to 100 hours or four days after you take it. The implications for build-up in the system are huge for people who take several pills a day for years. According to Professor Heather Ashton, 0.5 milligrams (mg) of Xanax, an often-prescribed benzodiazepine, is equivalent to 10 mg of Valium. Someone taking 6 mg of Xanax, which sounds like a relatively small dose, is taking the equivalent of 120 mg Valium, a huge dose. According to Jay Cohen, M.D., "The shorter the half-life, the more addictive the drug."

Benzodiazepines And GABA

Neurotransmitters are classified as either excitatory or inhibitory. The inhibitory neurotransmitters function to inhibit or slow down excitatory messages to the brain and nervous system. GABA is the most widely distributed neurotransmitter, present in concentrations of 200 to 1000 times greater than other neurotransmitters such as acetylcholine, norepinephrine, and serotonin. GABA is needed in the GABA receptors, not benzodiazepines.

GABA (Gamma Amino Butyric Acid), an amino acid, functions as an inhibitory neurotransmitter in the brain, and is what belongs in the GABA receptors. GABA is called the anxiety amino acid as it inhibits anxiety, fear, panic, alcohol addiction, and depression. GABA inhibits or slows down the firing of anxiety and panic-related messages at the decision-making part of the brain known as the cortex. GABA fills the group of receptor sites that slow down and block excitatory messages, so the cortex is not overwhelmed with anxiety, panic, pain or craving.

During times of stress the body can become depleted of necessary neurotransmitters causing one to feel anxious and fearful. Benzodiazepines act by filling the GABA receptor sites. GABA receptors are located in the brain and throughout the body. Because of this wide disbursement of receptors, benzodiazepines not only affect the brain, but the whole body as well.

Benzodiazepine use actually suppresses the production of the natural calming neurotransmitters as well as reducing the amount of other neurotransmitters including norepinephrine, serotonin, acetylcholine, and dopamine. These neurotransmitters are necessary for normal alertness, memory, muscle tone and coordination, emotional responses, endocrine gland secretions, heart rate, and blood pressure. As Peter Breggin states in his book *Brain Disabling Treatments in Psychiatry*; "At present, there are no known biochemical imbalances in the brain of typical psychiatric patients—until they are given psychiatric drugs."

Long-term use of benzodiazepines causes many side effects, including poor memory and cognition, emotional blunting, depression, increased anxiety, and dependence. Benzodiazepine use seems to both *cause and aggravate depression*. The depression is probably due to the decrease of neurotransmitters such as serotonin and norepinephrine.

Evidence suggests benzodiazepines are no longer effective after a few weeks of regular use. As tolerance to the drug develops one will begin to experience withdrawal symptoms between doses even though the drug is still being taken. Benzodiazepines suppress the production of natural calming neurotransmitters *causing* the most prominent symptom of withdrawal...increased anxiety.

Withdrawing From Benzodiazepines

There are many good reasons to stop using benzodiazepines. *Psychiatric Annals* (Vol. 25, No. 3. March 1995
p. 171) states; "The benzodiazepine-treated patients appeared to be better off and less symptomatic from anxiety
and depression when free of benzodiazepines." Many
people, after withdrawing from benzodiazepines, have
said they realized their daily operating levels were below
par during all the years of usage. Recall that long-term
use of benzodiazepines actually becomes the cause of anxiety and depression; you cannot get better until you stop
using them. *Use extreme caution when starting any drug
withdrawal program. Do not begin withdrawal unless you
follow a program that advises you how and what to do and
what to expect. Your nutritional support program should
be in place prior to withdrawal to restore needed brain
nutrients.*

The most important thing to remember after you decide to withdraw from any benzodiazepine is ***do not stop
suddenly,*** especially if you have been taking them for any

Xanax Taper			
Example: Patient taking 3 mg of Alprazolam (Xanax) per day.			
Week Number	Dose per Day (mg)	Week Number	Dose per Day (mg)
1	2.75	7	1.25
2	2.50	8	1.00
3	2.25	9	0.75
4	2.00	10	0.50
5	1.75	11	0.25
6	1.50	12	Off

Source: *Psychiatric Annals*, March 1995

length of time. *You must taper off slowly* and provide your body with a proper nutritional support program to be successful. It can take anywhere from several months to a year to completely stop benzodiazepines.

People will often try to abstain from or come off their drug too quickly, leaving them with the feeling of failure and the fear they will never be able to discontinue the drug. Symptoms of abrupt withdrawal are wide ranging and include anxiety, irritability, weight loss, chills, muscle weakness, tremors, apathy, craving for the medication, dizziness, nightmares, anger, rage, stomachaches, intestinal cramps, flu-like symptoms, restlessness, increased sensitivity to noise, light, touch, or smell, insomnia, convulsions, depression, hallucinations, vomiting, muscle cramping, and pain. These symptoms are greatly reduced and become quite tolerable when supported nutritionally and withdrawal is done slowly.

We cannot stress enough the importance of a good nutritional support program. Long-term benzodiazepine

Benzodiazepine Withdrawal Table
Valium (Diazepam) 20 mg, 2.5 mg tablets

Week	Morning	Lunch	Evening	Total	Mg Total
1.	2½ tabs	2 tabs	2½ tabs =	7 tabs	17½ mg
2.	2 tabs	2 tabs	2 tabs =	6 tabs	15 mg
3.	1½ tabs	1½ tabs	1½ tabs =	5 tabs	12½ mg
4.	1 tab	1½ tabs	1½ tab =	4 tabs	10 mg
5.	1 tab	1 tab	1 tab =	3 tabs	7½ mg
6.	½ tab	½ tab	1 tab =	2 tabs	5 mg
7.	½ tab		½ tab =	1 tab	2½ mg
8.			½ tab =	½ tab	1¼ mg
9.	off				

Use this schedule for withdrawal from most of the benzodiazepines. *Reduce by no more than one-fourth the daily dosage per 7 days!*

use takes over the body's own natural tranquilizer system, and as a result, GABA receptor sites in the brain reduce in number and the production of GABA decreases. Other neurotransmitters in the brain decrease as well, leaving the brain with little defense against anxiety, and depression. A nutritional support program using amino acids helps the brain to recover its natural functions by replacing and replenishing the neurotransmitters and their receptor sites.

The best way to withdraw is to begin tapering your dose. The drug detoxification handbooks used in most psychiatric hospitals recommend a dose reduction of one-fourth (¼th) the daily dose per 7 days. *Be sure to start the nutritional support program one week before you begin tapering off the drug.* Never compare the number

Phenobarbital Withdrawal Conversion For Benzodiazepines

Benzodiazepine	Dose (mg)	Phenobarbital Withdrawal Conversion (mg)
Alprazolam (Xanax)	0.5-1.0	30
Chlordiazepoxide (Librium)	25	30
Clonazepam (Klonopin)	2	30
Chlorazepate (Tranxene)	15	30
Diazepam (Valium)	0	30
Flurazepam (Dalmane)	30	30
Lorazepam (Ativan)	2	30
Temazepam (Restoril)	15	30
Triazolam (Halcion)	.25-0.50	30
Quazepam (Doral)	15	30
Estazolam (ProSom)	2	30

Source: *Psychiatric Annals*, March 1995

of milligrams; 1 mg of one drug cannot be substituted for 1 mg of another drug. For example, 5 mg of Valium does not equal 5 mg of Halcion or 5 mg of Ativan. Remember, these guidelines are just that—guidelines, nothing more. You might need to taper more slowly, staying on a dose for two weeks rather than one. The most important thing to remember is to keep moving forward. *Do not go backward by increasing doses again.*

Nutritional Support For Benzodiazepine Withdrawal

Long-term benzodiazepine use reduces all of the major neurotransmitters in the brain. A total neurotransmitter and vitamin complex such as Brain Link helps to restore them, or if you prefer capsules, use Super BNC (Super Balanced Neurotransmitter Complex).

If you suffer from stress and anxiety, chances are you are magnesium deficient. Magnesium helps control anxiety. At the Pain & Stress Center we use magnesium chloride form as Mag Link (capsules) or Mag Chlor 85 (liquid). Magnesium helps GABA to function and reach the receptor sites in the brain. Magnesium is essential to your recovery.

An omega 3 essential fatty acid (EFA) such as ProDHA provides support for the brain and nervous system. Studies show EFAs improve mood and play a major role with depression.

Anxiety Control is a balanced formula containing the amino acids (GABA, glycine, and glutamine); two calming herbs (Passion Flower and Primula Officinalis); and the co-factors, B-6 and magnesium. Anxiety Control is very effective in reducing anxiety safely and naturally.

L–T® (L-Theanine), a free-form amino acid found in green tea leaves, produces a tranquilizing effect in the brain without causing drowsiness or dull feelings. Studies reflect L-T increases alpha waves in the brain that promote muscle relaxation, and decrease stress-tension pain. You can use Anxiety Control between doses of L–T, if you feel overly stressed. For faster action, open the capsules and dissolve in water or juice.

Mood Sync* contains 5-HTP and amino acids that increase your serotonin and dopamine levels restoring the brain chemistry, alleviating depression, and mood swings. According to *Psychiatric Annals* (Vol. 25, No. 3, March 1995, p. 176) it states, "Depression is a consistent feature of benzodiazepine withdrawal."

Alpha KG and citric acid are components of the Krebs cycle, the chemical engine generating energy for every cell in the body. Fatigue is often a real issue when withdrawing off any drug. Alpha KG supports increased stamina and energy.

Taurine is the second most prevalent inhibitory neurotransmitter in the brain. Taurine reduces muscle pain, tremors, and shaking.

Liquid Serotonin under your tongue gives you a boost of serotonin to help you get through a stressful moment or situation.

Insomnia is a common problem for many as they withdraw from benzodiazepines. In *Psychiatric Annals* (Vol. 25, No. 3, March 1995, p 176), it states, "Benzodiazepines disrupt normal sleep patterns, suppressing slow wave sleep, rapid eye movement sleep, and dreaming. It may take several months to reestablish a normal sleep pattern

*CAUTION: DO NOT use if you are currently taking an SSRI (such as Prozac), MAO, or tricyclic antidepressant. If you are taking medications, and you don't know whether you are taking one of the drugs, ask your pharmacist.

when discontinued."

Sleep in vitally important to help you recover. At the Pain & Stress Center, we use Sleep Link or 5-HTP along with Mag Chlor at bedtime. If you are unable to sleep, you can add a capsule of Mellow Mind (Ashwagandha).

Daily Nutritional Support For Benzodiazepine Withdrawal

Mood Sync® – 1 or 2 morning and afternoon.

Anxiety Control – 2 three times per day.

Rodex B6 (150 mg timed release) - 1 in morning.

Mag Link® – 2 twice to three times per day, divided. Dosage should be adjusted to individual's bowel tolerance. If loose stools or diarrhea occur, decrease by 1 capsule, or try spacing further apart. *OR* **Mag Chlor** – can be used instead of Mag Link. Take 10 to 25 drops (one dropper full), two to three times per day.

Decaf Green Tea Extract – 1 capsule, two times daily.

Brain Link Complex* – 2 to 3 scoops in morning in juice, or 2 SBNC (Super Balanced Neurotransmitter Complex*) capsules, twice in the morning and afternoon.

L-T® (L-Theanine Complex) – 2 capsules, twice daily.

Taurine – 1 (1000 mg) capsule, twice daily for tremors and shaking.

Liquid Serotonin – 10 to 15 drops as needed, throughout the day for acute anxiety or nervousness.

B Complex – 1 in morning.

Sleep Link® – 1 or 2 capsules, 30 minutes before bedtime, or you can use 2, 5-HTP 50 mg capsules, 30 minutes

*CAUTION: DO NOT use if you are currently taking an SSRI (such as Prozac), MAO, or tricyclic antidepressant. If you are taking medications, and you don't know whether you are taking one of the drugs, ask your pharmacist.

prior to bedtime.

Mellow Mind** – 1 capsule (500 mg Ashwagandha) at bedtime, if needed in addition to Sleep Link.

Exercise such as walking, swimming, golf, or tennis daily.

IMPORTANT NOTE
About Nutritional Program
You may not need all of the supplements listed.
The supplements listed are only guidelines.

The minimum nutritional support would be Brain Link, ProDHA and Mag Chlor 85. Add in other supplements based on the symptoms you are experiencing.

For example, start with the first three suggested products. If you are having additional anxiety, add in the Anxiety Control, L-Theanine, *or* Liquid Serotonin. If you can't sleep use the nutritional support products listed for insomnia.

The same reduction schedule can be used for any dosage. Reduce the amount you take by one-fourth (¼th) the total dosage per week.

The time frames for these withdrawal schedules are *guidelines only.* You may find you need to spend two weeks on a reduced amount; this is fine. Just remember to keep coming down on the amount you are taking. Once you have reduced your dose, do not increase again to a higher amount. You are better to stabilize at lower dose than acclimate to the higher one again. *Some people who*

***CAUTION:** DO NOT use if you are currently taking an SSRI (such as Prozac), MAO, or tricyclic antidepressant. If you are taking medications, and you don't know whether you are taking one of the drugs, ask your pharmacist.

****CAUTION:** DO NOT use if taking any benzodiazepine.

have taken benzodiazepines for a number of years will take as long as six months to a year to stop completely. The last dose seems to be the hardest for people to give up. By the time you have reduced down to 1/8 mg per day completely stopping is a very small step.

Just do it! Then is when your freedom really begins!

Other Helpful Tips

If you are withdrawing from benzodiazepines, do not take Ambien a commonly prescribed sleeping pill. Although Ambien is not a benzodiazepine, it works by affecting the GABA receptors in much the same way the benzodiazepines do and will be counterproductive.

Daily exercise such as walking, swimming, cycling, golf, tennis, or any physical activity you enjoy and will do is important at this time. Exercise reduces anxiety and will elevate endorphin levels in the brain. Deep breathing and meditation or relaxation exercises will help to relax you and can change the brain chemistry.

Withdrawal symptoms are a sign that your body is healing. Benzodiazepines cause emotional blunting, this means that you have not been experiencing normal pleasure or pain. As your body begins to detoxify normal feelings begin to emerge. This might feel overwhelming at first because you are not used to experiencing feelings. As you learn to just accept your feelings, both good and bad, you will realize what it feels like to be truly alive.

Psychological support as you withdraw is very important. Benzodiazepines cause emotional blunting, and coming off them will allow long suppressed feelings to emerge. A good counselor or therapist can help you deal with these issues and resolving them brings true healing. Emotional support from your spouse, partner, or good friend is important. This person must educate him or herself about benzodiazepine withdrawal to help you through this tough time.

Some physicians recommend switching drugs to help with withdrawal. For example, if you have been taking a medium acting benzodiazepine such as Xanax, they will recommend changing to Valium, a longer acting drug. However, all benzodiazepines have the same actions and a longer acting drug continues to decrease the normal neurotransmitter function in the brain as well as prolonging the addiction. Amino acids help heal the brain, and leave you better prepared to live drug free.

Most importantly, remember that withdrawal symptoms will not last forever. They will pass and you will have your freedom from prescribed drugs. Take one day at a time and remember this problem did not happen in one day. Be patient with yourself—this too will pass.

4
Prozac, The Beginning
Of SSRI Drugs

When doctors prescribe psychiatric drugs for depression, they often tell their patients depression is caused by a chemical imbalance in the brain, and a SSRI (Selective Serotonin Reuptake Inhibitor) drug will resolve this imbalance. Glaxo Smith Kline, the manufacturers of Paxil, run television ads saying the same thing, "Depression *may* be caused by a chemical imbalance in the brain."

Peter Breggin, M.D., author of *Brain Disabling Treatments in Psychiatry* states, "At present, there are no known biochemical imbalances in the brain of typical psychiatric patients—until they are given psychiatric drugs." In other words, psychiatric drugs *cause* chemical imbalances in the brain. They *do not cure* this supposed imbalance, nor do they cure depression. They only block symptoms. Peter Breggin, M.D., author of *Talking Back To Prozac*, states, "Prozac is much more potent than caffeine and your brain is far more vulnerable and easily damaged than your computer. Taking Prozac, in summary constitutes a toxic interference in the brain. If it feels good, it means you prefer impaired brain function to normal brain function."

Prozac (Fluoxetine) was the first of a class of drugs known as SSRIs or Selective Serotonin Reuptake Inhibitors. Eli Lilly began marketing Prozac in 1988 and it soon became the wonder drug of the '90s. Prozac, within two years of its appearance on the market, became the number one prescribed antidepressant. Other drug companies got on the SSRI bandwagon. Pfizer introduced Zoloft in 1992. Paxil was released by Glaxo Smith Kline in 1993. Today, there are multiple SSRI drugs on the market. Besides the original three, (Prozac, Zoloft, and Paxil) there are Effexor, Luvox, Serzone, Celexa, Lexapro, and Wellbutrin. Sarafem, a drug prescribed to women for PMS symptoms is actually Prozac distributed under a new name for marketing purposes. Serzone and Wellbutrin are not true SSRIs as they affect other neurotransmitters in the brain besides serotonin. But we listed them here because they do block the reuptake of serotonin. Zyban, a drug prescribed to help with smoking cessation is Wellbutrin with a new marketing twist, but all the same nasty side effects.

In March 1990, Prozac made it on the cover of News Week with the headline, *The Promise of Prozac*. In this glowing review, Prozac was described as a *medical breakthrough* already being prescribed for so many conditions besides depression that even "healthy people have started asking for it." The problem with a healthy person starting on these drugs is that once SSRIs are started they are very hard to stop. SSRIs have a long list of side effects, some of which can be permanently disabling. Drug companies state SSRIs are not habit forming. Yet in the *Physicians' Desk Reference* all the SSRI drugs listed state no studies have been performed to evaluate the effects of long-term use. Despite the *non-habit forming* marketing campaign, people who try to stop taking SSRIs suffer a wide range of withdrawal symptoms. The withdrawal symptoms often force many individuals to remain on a drug they really don't need. In fact, there is potential for brain damage with long-term use. Glaxo Smith Kline, the manufacturer of Paxil, is currently in the midst of a class action suit for their statement claiming Paxil is not habit-forming.

Jay S. Cohen, M.D., in his book *Over Dose* refers to a study in the *Journal of Clinical Psychiatry* stating nearly 85% of people treated with Prozac complain of diarrhea, 70% suffer profuse sweating, and 32% get headaches. An additional 22 to 34% of patients taking Prozac, developed insomnia, and required additional medication for sleep. About 40% of senior citizens require sleep medication to control Prozac-induced insomnia. Prozac's listed side effects are the same symptoms shown in Serotonin Syndrome that occur when someone has too much serotonin. Dr. Cohen makes the point in his book that drug companies manufacture dose sizes based on an average weight of 170 pounds. Even the smallest dose available will probably be too much for those weighing less than 170 pounds. According to Dr. Cohen's research most patients taking Prozac get 100 to 400% more than they needed for effective treatment.

In 1993 Peter Kramer, M.D., a psychiatrist, wrote *Listening to Prozac*. Dr. Kramer makes sensational claims about the benefits of Prozac. He insists the drug not only treats serious depression but also cures everyday maladies such as shyness, sensitivity, low self-esteem, jealousy, fear of intimacy, fear of rejection, perfectionism, fastidiousness, lack of confidence, and competiveness; conditions that have long been addressed with psychotherapy. According to Dr. Kramer, with the advent of Prozac there is no need to see a therapist to work on personal issues, the miracle drug Prozac cures you of personal character flaws and you become the wonderful person you had always wanted to be—confident, balanced, loving, secure and bold with the ingestion of one simple, safe pill; a miracle drug. It is natural to assume this drug is perfectly safe. After all, it was approved by the Federal Drug Administration (FDA), and it is prescribed by your doctor who is knowledgeable of all medications. He would never recommend anything that is not in your absolute best interest.

Let's take a closer look at pharmaceutical industry and learn why our assumption of protection from the FDA and our doctors is wrong. Doctors are given information from the drug companies. More specifically their sales representatives' sole responsibility is to convince the doctor to prescribe their new wonder drug.

Pharmaceutical Companies, The FDA And Doctors

People assume an FDA approved medication is safe, but what the FDA is really saying is the benefits outweigh the risks, *not that there are no risks.* The truth of the matter is drugs have side effects. If you read the *Physicians' Desk Reference,* most drugs have long lists of potential side effects. Some of them are pretty scary. Although the tide is changing, many of us are overly trusting when our doctors make recommendations for medications. Currently, the use of these drugs is increasing in younger and younger children. This is a frightening trend to us at the Pain & Stress Center.

Drug companies have the largest lobby in Washington. They contribute huge amounts of money to political campaigns, and that makes them a powerful influence with our elected officials. The FDA receives half its budget for the evaluation of new drugs from drug company user's fees. This makes the agency financially dependent on the industry it regulates—an obvious conflict of interest.

While the FDA has considerable staff to work towards approving new drugs the staff allocated to monitor harmful side effects is insufficient. Once the FDA approves a drug and dangerous side effects begin to emerge it takes years before any action is taken to either warn of these side effects or remove it from the market.

A horrifying example of a dangerous drug getting to and remaining on the market is Rezulin, a drug prescribed for type II diabetics. Dr. John Gueriguian, the FDA officer evaluating Rezulin, voiced concerns about the drug's potential for damage to the liver and heart. After Warner-Lambert executives protested, Gueriguian was removed from the evaluation process and replaced. Rezulin was soon approved for general use in the spring of 1997. By October 1997, the FDA was already receiving reports of severe liver failure due to this drug. By December 1997, only a few months after its approval, there had been six Rezulin-related deaths. At this point British officials withdrew Rezulin from use in England. The FDA did not follow their example; Rezulin continued to be prescribed in the United States until March 1998. By the time Rezulin was pulled off the market sixty-three deaths had been confirmed from it's use. Rezulin remained on the market for three years and yet within three months of it's launching the FDA knew this was a lethal drug. So much for assuming protection from the FDA!

Many people think the FDA performs the tests and studies on drugs to prove their safety. However, drug manufacturers conduct all the testing; they only submit final test results to the FDA for review. Drug companies are very involved with the researchers who test drugs in human subjects. In their contracts with academic researchers they insist on controlling how the research is done, how it is reported, or if it is to be reported at all.

The researchers are financially dependent on the funds the drug companies provide for research. This is another blatant conflict of interest.

Peter Breggin, M.D., reported the studies used to get approval for Prozac were woefully inadequate, and run poorly by individuals who had financial conflicts of interest. There were numerous irregularities; more studies failed than succeeded and the final results had to be reworked several times in order to make them acceptable. In the final analysis, the studies used for FDA approval included a mere 286 individuals who were exposed to Prozac for a maximum of six weeks, even though the drug is often prescribed indefinitely.

There have been several widely publicized instances of drug companies suppressing unfavorable research results. No long-term studies of SSRIs and their effects in the brain and body have been done. Dr. Breggin's research established SSRIs said to enhance serotonergic neurotransmission, grossly impair the process of neurotransmission. Prozac introduces a toxic interference in the brain.

Let's examine the relationship between our doctors and drug companies. In the year 2000 drug companies spent more than 8 billion dollars on gifts, meals, and trips to influence doctors to prescribe their drugs. The companies also fund much of the continuing medical education doctors need to renew their licenses. The information doctors know about a drug is what the drug company's sales representative tells him during sales calls, through seminars paid for, or sponsored by that same drug company. Another resource is a book called the *Physicians' Desk Reference (PDR)*. The *PDR* is considered the ultimate authority on every drug available. However, this reference is provided by the pharmaceutical companies. And as if all this wasn't enough to secure the drug companies place in the market, they spend several billion more dollars yearly marketing directly to us, the consumers. With all the drug ads on television today, many people go to their doctors requesting the drug they saw advertised last night on TV. In a recent survey, a large number of doctors said they often prescribe drugs based on patients' requests.

We expect the FDA and our doctors to protect us. Sadly, both are financially involved with or even dependent on the pharmaceutical companies that research, manufacture and market the drugs. *These companies are the most profitable in the world.* Dr. Marcia Angell, former editor-in-chief of the *New England Journal of Medicine* made the statement, "To rely on the drug companies for unbiased evaluations of their products makes about as much sense as relying on beer companies to teach us about alcoholism."

SSRI Drugs Negative Affects On the Brain

Doctors casually and frequently prescribe SSRI drugs, often with inadequate follow-up. It is known that antidepressants can cause mania and aggression in some people with the possibility of leading to acts of violence. The American Psychiatric Association's *Diagnostic and Statistical Manual of Mental Disorders, Fourth Edition (DSM-IV) (1994)* clearly states that all antidepressants can cause mania.

A man in Boston, Massachusetts got up from his desk, calmly walked in the Human Resources Department of his Internet software company and shot seven people to death. Reports that he was on an antidepressant drug should not come as a surprise. Fred A. Baughman, Jr. M.D., author of *The History of the Fraud of Biological Psychiatry* states, "Virtually every violent mass murder scene in recent years has been the result of individuals on Prozac, Zoloft, Paxil, or one of the other SSRI drugs". The school shooting in Littleton, Colorado involved a student on Luvox. The comedian, Phil Hartman, was murdered by his wife after she started taking Zoloft. The Atlanta day trader who killed his family and others before killing himself, was found with Prozac. There are a number of cases of parents, while on these drugs, killing their children and themselves in the most violent ways. Prozac alone has been involved in 2,500 deaths most by suicide or violence.

The brain is by far the most complex organ of the body; its mechanisms and actions in relation to thought and behavior are simply not known with certainty. Joseph Le Doux, author of *Synaptic Self*, believes the synapses, the spaces between neurons, are the true creators of who we are; what we think, how we act, what we feel, our personality traits, preferences and beliefs. SSRI drugs directly impact the synapses that Le Doux says make each of us an individual. Fred A. Baughman, Jr., MD, a highly respected neurologist and expert in the field, postulates that statements of chemical imbalances causing problems are just theories. There is no scientific evidence that a person with depression or anxiety has a chemical imbalance. The imbalance occurs when you take psychiatric drugs.

Drugs like Prozac work by interfering with the metabolism of the brain. Serotonin crosses the synaptic gap and travels from one neuron to another. Once serotonin activates the neuron, the brain reabsorbs the leftover chemical. The function of an SSRI is to prevent reabsorption, allowing serotonin to remain in the synapse and interact with its targets for a prolonged time. The extended exposure to serotonin is not necessary and is what causes the brain to start making adaptations such as reducing the sensitivity to serotonin as well as the number of serotonin receptor sites. SSRIs like Prozac do more than just block serotonin reuptake; they stimulate the release of vast amounts of serotonin from the nerve endings into the brain. Scientists believe that the large amount of serotonin could cause extensive brain damage. Brain imbalances exist as either excesses or deficiencies of neurotransmitters.

Talk of brain abnormalities causing mental illness is simply theory never scientifically proven. Dr. Baughman has carefully studied research indicating that brain abnormalities cause mental illnesses like ADHD (Attention Deficit Hyperactivity Disorder). Dr. Baughman believes these studies actually prove *psychiatric drugs* cause brain abnormalities since the *only individuals with the brain abnormalities are those who have been on the drugs prescribed for treatment.* As amazing as this may sound, the concept of chemical imbalances and brain abnormalities causing mental illness has been talked about over the years to the point it is accepted as true. This concept has been promoted because it creates a huge market for companies and industries claiming to have a drug supposedly capable of fixing the imbalance or abnormality. The market for such drugs is in the billions of dollars.

Neurotransmitters

Neurotransmitters are the chemical messengers or language in the brain. There are more than 100 known neurotransmitters, but only about 10 are used for communication between brain cells. Different neurotransmitters carry different messages in the brain; some carry pain sensations, while others carry voluntary muscle movement; some cause excitatory emotional responses, while others are inhibitory in nature. Our reactions to *everything* we encounter, the way we are stirred by a song, angered by an argument, experience hurt from emotional pain caused by a loved one, or feel the joy of friendship—every emotion we feel is dependent on neurotransmitters.

Candace Pert Ph.D. refers to neurotransmitters as the molecules of emotion. Too many or too few neurotransmitters will cause you to under or overreact depending on the stimulus. Neurotransmitters work in concert with each other; changing the level of one affects others. The four main neurotransmitters that concern us in reference to the SSRI drugs are serotonin, dopamine, norepinephrine, and adrenaline. These are often referred to as *the feel good* neurotransmitters. Antidepressant drugs will usually target one or more of these neurotransmitters.

Brain cells communicate using neurotransmitters. When serotonin is released from the sending cell, it travels across a microscopic distance called a synapse to the receiving cell. Once a signal has been sent, the sending brain cell will clean up any unused serotonin through a process called *reuptake*. Reuptake ensures that lingering serotonin will not continue to stimulate the receiving cell. That is where the SSRI drugs do their work, at the reuptake channels.

Selective Serotonin Reuptake Inhibitors or SSRIs block the serotonin reuptake channels, leaving all the excess serotonin that normally would have been reabsorbed, to continue stimulating the receiving cell. This over-stimulation causes the brain to make compensatory changes to adapt to the increased levels of circulating serotonin. This adapted state cannot be defined as normal. By blocking reuptake, the body's natural recycling process is short-circuited. This exacerbates existing deficiencies.

Changes in natural systems often cause unexpected reactions. It was originally thought that wearing a back brace all the time would lessen the occurrence of back injuries in normal people performing certain types of work. In fact, this practice caused a weakening of the muscles that normally support the back and resulted in more injuries. Likewise, increasing the level of serotonin the way SSRI drugs do has shown in animal studies to cause compensation that reduces the production of serotonin receptor sites. These studies show receptor sites are lost permanently, indicating permanent brain damage. Peter Breggin, M.D., commented, "Neither the FDA, nor any of the drug companies, are interested in studying this issue."

Today, sixteen years after the advent of Prozac, scientists have a much greater understanding of neurotransmitters and how they function. They now know that only about 5% of the serotonin in the body is found in the brain. The other 95% is found throughout the body—in the gastrointestinal tract, in the cardiovascular system, in blood cells, in the reproductive organs. It plays a significant role in controlling a host of hormones that regulate a multitude of physiologic processes. Research scientists also know neurotransmitters do not work independently of each other. When you artificially change the levels of one neurotransmitter, others change to try to regain a semblance of balance. They have found overstimulating receptor sites, such as in the case of someone on an SSRI drug, causes the receptors to become desensitized over time. Once receptor sites become desensitized, the brain cannot function without the higher levels of circulating serotonin. This explains why people usually plummet

Prozac Precautions

Major Symptom Warnings

Anxiety and insomnia

Altered appetite and weight

Activation of mania

Seizures

Suicide

Headaches

Tremor

Nausea

Interference with Cognitive and Motor Performance

"Any psychoactive drug may impair judgment, thinking, or motor skills, and patients should be cautioned about operating hazardous machinery, including automobiles, until they are reasonably certain that the drug treatment does not affect them adversely."

Impairment of Fertility
(Paraphrased for brevity)

In studies performed using rats and rabbits, there were no adverse effects on fertility. However, in rat studies there was an increase in stillborn pups, a decrease in birth weight, and an increase in deaths during the first seven days postpartum. Prozac should be used during pregnancy, only if the potential benefits justify the potential risks.

Nursing Mothers

Prozac is excreted in human milk, nursing while on Prozac is not recommended.

Pediatric Use

Safety and effectiveness in pediatric patients has not been established.

Source: *Physicians' Desk Reference, 2002*

into depression, if they stop these drugs suddenly. This is not a true depression, but a reaction to withdrawal from the drug. Unfortunately, many doctors do not know or understand this withdrawal symptom, and immediately restart the patient on the drug. As with any dependency, continuing on the drug stops the withdrawal symptoms. However the harmful effects of the drug on the brain and body continue. Each time you stop, then start any drug, the withdrawal symptoms increase.

Side Effects

The point of concern is serotonin is found throughout the body and brain. Any drug affecting the levels of serotonin has a wide range of effects on the cardiovascular, gastrointestinal, reproductive and endocrine systems. Neurotransmitters do not act independently. When you artificially change the level of one neurotransmitter, changes take place in others as well. Serotonin and dopamine are closely linked. When you take an SSRI drug, it forces an increase of circulating serotonin that causes a compensatory drop in dopamine. When dopamine levels drop, acetylcholine activity increase.

Joseph Glenmullen, M.D., author of *Prozac Backlash*, states, "When disturbances to the dopamine/acetylcholine balance happens it can cause four different neurological side effects that have to do with loss of motor control. The side effects that have been consistently reported with the serotonin boosting drugs are: 1) facial tics, 2) muscle spasms that can be mild but may be so severe that the body becomes locked in bizarre positions know as tardive dyskinesia, 3) agitation, and 4) drug-induced Parkinson's disease."

Fatigue is one of the first symptoms of Parkinson's disease. People on SSRI drugs often complain about fatigue. Dr. Glenmullen hypothesizes that this fatigue experienced by patients taking an SSRI may be the first sign of drug-induced Parkinson's. Sometimes discontinuing the drug stops the side effects; but not always.

Candace B. Pert, Ph.D., the pharmacologist who discovered the opiate receptor in the brain, made this statement in "Letter to the Editor" in *TIME Magazine*, October 20, 1997, "I am alarmed at the monster that John Hopkins neuroscientist, Solomon Snyder, and I created when we discovered the simple binding assay for drug receptors 25 years ago. Prozac and other antidepressant serotonin-receptor-active compounds may also cause cardiovascular problems in some susceptible people after long-term use, which has become common practice despite the lack of safety studies."

"The public is being misinformed about the precision of these selective serotonin-reuptake inhibitors when the medical profession oversimplifies their action in the brain and ignores the body as if it exists merely to carry the head around! In short, these molecules of emotion regulate *every aspect* of our physiology. A new paradigm has evolved, with implications that life-style changes such as diet and exercise can offer profound, safe and natural mood elevation."

Lexapro, the newest SSRI to hit the market, has this precaution on its label under the heading abnormal bleeding, "Published case reports have documented the *occurrence of bleeding episodes in patients treated with psychotropic drugs that interfere with serotonin reuptake.* Subsequent epidemiological studies, both of the case-control and cohort design, have demonstrated an association between use of psychotropic drugs that interfere with serotonin reuptake and the occurrence of upper gastrointestinal bleeding. In two studies, concurrent use of a nonsteroidal anti-inflammatory drug (NSAIDs) or aspirin potentiated the risk of bleeding. Although these studies focused on upper gastrointestinal bleeding, there is reason to believe that bleeding at other sites may be similarly potentiated. Patients should be cautioned regarding the risk of bleeding associated with concomitant use of Lexapro with NSAIDs, aspirin, or other drugs that affect coagulation."

Reports of side effects from SSRI drugs began surfacing in psychiatric journals as early as 1991. The side effects emerging with serotonin boosters are consistent with those seen in the major tranquilizers of the 1950s, 1960s and 1970s. Thorazine was the first in this class of drugs that grew to include more than a dozen drugs. Within ten years of Thorazine's arrival in the market, there were many reports of neurological side effects. These same side effects are now being seen with SSRI drugs.

The major tranquilizers act by suppressing the dopamine level directly; SSRI drugs do it indirectly. The major tranquilizers, also called neuroleptics, have proven to alter normal activities in the brain. They can cause bizarre behavior and even permanent damage in what was, prior to the drugs, a normally functioning system. Tardive dyskinesia and dystonia are two symptoms you see as a result of SSRIs. TD is an abnormality that causes a person to have uncontrollable movements and spasms of muscles in the body or face. These uncontrollable twitches, spasms, and writhing movements are usually *permanent and irreversible*. TD occurs at the amazing rate of 5% per year for patients exposed to this particular class of drugs for 3 months or more. After five years of exposure, TD afflicts at least 25% of patients. Most long-term patients eventually develop this malady.

You've seen in movies or documentaries mental institution patients that with weird repetitive movements of body parts. They have tardive dyskinesia. They did not develop TD until drugs were implemented at the institution. *The very thing making them appear the most crazy is caused by the drugs!* Considering the occurrence of tardive dyskinesia and the ease of observing it, surely measures would be taken to warn of the dangers of these drugs? Patients received these drugs in the 1950s, but the FDA required no such warnings until 1985. Millions of people are now permanently afflicted with TD. It took the FDA 30 years to require a uniform warning for such an obvious, easily observable occurrence.

What did the drug companies and doctors prescribing these drugs say about the weird, uncontrollable movements? They said it was just part of the patients' mental illness. In other words, crazy people act weird. Today, when a person on an SSRI murders his friends and himself, they say depressed people do these things. You must ask the question if these drugs effectively treat depression, then why would they still be considered depressed? Is it just coincidence that these persons did not commit any acts of violence until *after* starting on medication?

More adverse reactions have been reported on Prozac than *any drug in history*. There have been 2,500 deaths related to Prozac's use—most due to suicide or violence. The drug companies manufacturing the SSRI drugs earn a combined income from these drugs of 6 billion dollars a year. They do not want you to know the truth about these drugs and their side effects.

History Should Be Remembered

Time and time again, a new drug is promoted as safe and effective. Manufacturers claim great results. Before long, terrible side effects and addiction or worse are the end result. Finally, after a long list of casualties, it becomes a controlled substance and an illegal street drug. Prescribed addiction!

Eric Harris 18, a student at Columbine High School in Colorado, shot and killed 13 people for no reason. Harris had undergone anger management treatments and was on the SSRI, Luvox. Harris had a therapeutic blood level of Luvox at the time of his autopsy. Kip Kinkel, 14, killed 2 and injured 22 during a shooting spree in Springfield, Oregon. Kinkel had been treated for anger and was on psychiatric drugs. Did these drugs control their urges to hurt others and take lives—definitely not!

The Bayer Company began producing Heroin in 1898. Heroin was supposed to be the safe alternative to Morphine. Eli Lilly, the maker of Prozac, also produced methadone and LSD. Later, Methadone was prescribed to get people off Heroin, but was just as addictive. LSD, initially produced for use by the CIA in mind control experiments, was promoted as being safe for psychiatric use. Eli Lilly introduced Darvon in 1957 and promoted it as non-addictive. Twenty years and many deaths later, warnings were finally required. In the late 1950s, Parke, Davis & Company introduced PCP (angel dust) as a painkiller. *Medical studies* had shown that PCP had a large margin of safety. Valium was supposed to be safe, then found to be very addictive. Xanax was introduced as a safer drug to replace Valium, but it turned out to be even *more addictive*. The same story goes for cocaine and amphetamines—once promoted as safe and effective, now controlled substances.

Summary

SSRI drugs cause an alteration in normal brain functioning. This alteration could be irreversible. Prozac, the first SSRI, had more adverse reaction reports than any drug in history. These adverse reactions include attempted suicide, violence, aggression, and paranoia. Over 2,500 deaths are associated with Prozac; most are due to suicide or violence. Recently, individuals on Prozac or other psychiatric drugs have committed horrendous mass murders.

The FDA, the regulatory agency involved in the approval of drugs like Prozac, does not adequately protect the public from dangerous drugs. Furthermore, members of the FDA involved in the drug approval process have personal financial conflicts of interest, work or receive monies for the companies that they are approving. Is this really objective?

Clinical trials for new drugs last only six to eight weeks and contain only a few hundred people. Yet when these medications become available, they are prescribed to millions of people who take them for years and years. No controlled studies exist for the long-term effects of SSRI drugs, despite the great need.

Recently, the National Institute of Health (NIH) Women's Health Initiative long-term health study was stopped due to the adverse side effects from Prempro. Prempro was a hormone replacement therapy for postmenopausal women to reduce the risk of heart disease and breast cancer. The study was scheduled to run for 8.5 years, but it was discontinued after only five years. Mounting evidence indicated the drug actually increased the risk for all the diseases it was being prescribed to prevent. Until this study, no long-term studies existed.

Similar long-term controlled studies desperately need to be conducted on the SSRI class of drugs. Harmful drugs have historically been introduced by drug companies and withdrawn only when faced with enough public outcries.

Natural Alternatives

The key to normal brain function is to put back in the brain what belongs there—not to suppress or increase the action of any neurotransmitter with chemicals. Amino acids and other nutrients are what the brain requires to function well. Amino acids and brain function go hand in hand. Amino acids create needed neurotransmitters. If you took all the fat and water out of the body 75% of what would be left would be amino acids. Drugs *DO NOT* create neurotransmitters, amino acids do. If a person has a low serotonin level, using an SSRI drug further depletes an exhausted system. SSRI drugs raise the circulating serotonin in an artificial way potentially causing permanent harm to your brain and body over extended use. The natural and safe way to increase serotonin in the brain is to use the amino acid 5-HTP. The body metabolizes 5-HTP into serotonin. 5-HTP can be found in Mood Sync, HTP10, and Teen Link. These formulas, used when needed, plus Super Balanced Neurotransmitter Complex taken on a daily basis will supply the brain with the amino acids it needs to function.

Two other very important neuro-nutrients are omega-3 essential fatty acids and B-6. Research shows the effectiveness of these two supplements in treating depression.

Coming Off Zoloft—A Case Study

Patsy, a 35-year-old teacher, had been on Zoloft for

eight years when she came to the Pain & Stress Center seeking help. Patsy had been prescribed Zoloft for depression following a painful divorce. She told us as the doctor started her on the drug she would report back that she didn't think it was helping with her depression and he would raise the dose. She continued to see the prescribing doctor for about a year. When we first talked to Patsy she was on 100 mg of Zoloft. She said she didn't think the drug had ever really been helpful in raising her mood;

SSRI Reduction Schedule

Week 1	Day 1 100 mg	Day 2 75 mg	Day 3 100 mg	Day 4 75 mg	Day 5 100 mg	Day 6 75 mg	Day 7 100 mg
Week 2	Day 8 75 mg	Day 9 75 mg	Day 10 100 mg	Day 11 75 mg	Day 12 75 mg	Day 13 100 mg	Day 14 75 mg
Week 3	Day 15 75 mg	Day 16 75 mg	Day 17 100 mg	Day 18 75 mg	Day 19 75 mg	Day 20 75 mg	Day 21 100 mg
Week 4	Day 22 75 mg	Day 23 75 mg	Day 24 75 mg	Day 25 75 mg	Day 26 75 mg	Day 27 75 mg	Day 28 75 mg
Week 5	Day 29 75 mg	Day 30 50 mg	Day 31 75 mg	Day 32 50 mg	Day 33 75 mg	Day 34 50 mg	Day 35 75 mg
Week 6	Day 36 50 mg	Day 37 50 mg	Day 35 75 mg	Day 36 50 mg	Day 37 50 mg	Day 38 75 mg	Day 39 50 mg
Week 7	Day 40 50 mg	Day 41 50 mg	Day 42 75 mg	Day 43 50 mg	Day 44 50 mg	Day 45 50 mg	Day 46 75 mg
Week 8	Day 47 50 mg	Day 48 50 mg	Day 49 50 mg	Day 50 50 mg	Day 51 50 mg	Day 52 50 mg	Day 53 50 mg
Week 9	Day 54 50 mg	Day 55 25 mg	Day 56 50 mg	Day 57 25 mg	Day 58 50 mg	Day 59 25 mg	Day 60 50 mg
Week 10	Day 61 25 mg	Day 62 25 mg	Day 63 50 mg	Continue →	→	→	

Follow this a sample reduction schedule for safe, slow withdraw. We have used this reduction schedule successfully at the Pain & Stress Center.

however every time she tried to stop taking it she suffered severe withdrawal symptoms. She felt forced to start it again due to the withdrawal symptoms—vertigo, feelings of electric zaps (shocks), and emotional instability.

In order to rebuild Patsy's depleted neurotransmitters and improve brain function, she started on a nutritional support program. The program included Brain Link, Tyrosine 850, Mag Chlor 85, ProDHA, Rodex B6, and Anxiety Control. She was taking 100 mg of Zoloft once a day; we suggested a schedule to begin reducing the Zoloft (see previous page).

After Patsy reduced her overall dose by 25 mg and stabilized at the lower dose for at least two weeks, she then followed the same reduction cycle for the next 25 mg. Patsy did very well with this reduction schedule until she got down to 50/25/25/50 mg per day. When she tried to extend 25 mg for two days and then back up to 50 mg, she felt depressed and noticed more withdrawal symptoms. We recommended going back to the 50/25/50/25 schedule for another two weeks, and then try to extend the 25 mg to two days. This worked well for Patsy.

After Patsy had reduced her dose to 25 mg, we started her on HTP10, a low dose formula containing 10 mg of 5-HTP. This allowed her brain to produce more serotonin, but not so much that it created a conflict with the Zoloft. It took Patsy eight months to completely stop taking the Zoloft. After Patsy had stopped the Zoloft for 72 hours, she added the Mood Sync, in addition to what she was already taking. By using this slow reduction schedule, Patsy was able to successfully stop Zoloft.

5
The SSRI Story

Selective serotonin reuptake inhibitors (SSRIs) are not the magic bullets the drug companies would like you to believe they are. They all have multiple adverse side effects that influence the way you think, feel, and act.

SSRIs were designed to block the removal of the neurotransmitter serotonin from the brain synapse. Blocking reuptake causes an increased firing of serotonin nerves; this is an attempt to trick the brain into thinking it has more serotonin than it does. Serotonin is the master controller in the brain as it influences levels of the other neurotransmitters. It is manufactured in the brain from the amino acid, tryptophan, or more directly from 5-HTP (5-Hydroxytryptophan). SSRIs do not provide the raw materials necessary for the brain to produce more serotonin and by blocking the reuptake vesicles they stop the brain's natural recycling ability. The net effect of these drugs is to further deplete serotonin levels that are already low.

Research has documented many people taking SSRIs never improve; instead, they have increased anxiety, depression, agitation, insomnia and weight gain. According to Peter Breggin, M.D. Prozac, an SSRI, grossly impairs the process of neurotransmission and disrupts the brain's normal activity. As Dr. Breggin's research indicates, taking Prozac or any of the other SSRI drugs, introduces a toxic interference into the brain; this is due to drug induced emotional blunting or euphoria.

In March 2004 the FDA requested drug companies

change the label on ten widely used antidepressants including all SSRIs, to include warnings for the increased possibility of suicide. Of major concern is the effect on the brains of children and teens. SSRIs can spark agitation and impulsive acts that can lead to suicide attempts; children are more susceptible to this effect. Why is the FDA just *now* taking action to require these label warnings? According to Peter Breggin, M.D. and Jay Cohen, M.D., it is common knowledge that antidepressant drugs can induce mania. The DSM-IV, the diagnostic bible of psychiatric disorders, makes multiple references to the fact that antidepressants can cause mania.

The use of SSRI antidepressants in children has soared over the past few years with more than 1 million prescriptions for children and teens being filled. This rise has occurred even though the vast majority of clinical trials have failed to prove the medications are helpful in depressed children. Paradoxically, drugs that have never shown benefits for depressed children have some of the largest increases in prescription rates. Pediatric prescriptions for Paxil doubled between 1998 and 2002, despite the fact it failed to show it was any better than placebo in three different trials. In the March 2004 *FDA Letter*, it states, "Among antidepressants, only Prozac (fluoxetine) is approved for the treatment of pediatric major depressive disorder. Prozac (fluoxetine), Zoloft (sertraline), and Luvox (fluvoxamine) are approved for pediatric obsessive-compulsive disorder. None of these drugs are approved as monotherapy for use in treating bipolar depression, either in adults or children."

The story of Matthew, a 13 year-old boy, is a classic example of the damage that can be done by giving SSRIs to teens. After a family move Matthew was having trouble adjusting in a new school. The counselor suggested he see a psychiatrist. His parents complied and at the conclusion of the doctor's visit he was given an SSRI antidepressant to take. His parents reported the medication made him fidgety and restless. The morning after Matthew took his seventh pill his mother found him hanging by a belt from a laundry hook in his closet. His parents were not provided a package insert with prescribing information because the doctor gave them samples and set the dose. An autopsy revealed Matthew's body had SSRI levels that would be given to a 250-pound person. Matthew weighed less than 100 pounds. This is only one example of a child being hurt by SSRIs.

Obviously, there was gross negligence on the part of the prescribing physician, who as a psychiatrist, should have been better informed about dosing and should have known to warn patients of possible adverse side effects. But it seems the drug companies have done such a good job marketing SSRIs that everyone, doctors included, fail to look at them as the powerful psychiatric drugs they are. There have been no long-term studies to reflect the safety of SSRI drugs in children.

On August 22, 2003 the manufacturer of Effexor issued a *Dear Doctor* letter warning of the increased risk of "hostility and suicide-related adverse events, such as suicidal ideation and self harm in children age six to seventeen". Joseph Glenmullen, M.D., a Harvard psychiatrist, reported in his best selling book *Prozac Backlash*, that as early as 1990, two Harvard psychiatrists, reported that Prozac could induce "intense violent suicidal preoccupation." Dr. Glenmullen's book documents the dark side of SSRIs and their long list of dangerous side effects.

The FDA has finally requested drug label changes that warn of potentially dangerous side effects. The FDA action is intended to protect adults and children, but especially the potential of possible harm to children, teens, and younger. Jay Cohen, M.D. in an article posted on his web site, www.MedicationSense.com, states this action from the FDA is 16 years overdue. He further comments many doctors do not know how to properly prescribe antidepressants. Drug company sales reps have vigorously pushed antidepressants at family practitioners, pediatricians, and gynecologists, physicians who are not typically trained in the complex prescribing of antidepressant drugs. Consumers are inundated with television commercials that leave the impression antidepressant drugs are the perfect solution for a happy life.

Dr. Glenmullen wrote about the 10-20-30 year pattern typically seen in the life of psychiatric drugs. Initially, the drug company markets a new drug as being revolutiionary breakthrough for the treatment of depression, and far superior to predecessor drugs. The new drug moves out of the realms of psychiatry and begins to be prescribed by general practitioners for any number of maladies. After about ten years on the market problems begin to surface with the drug, which the drug manufacturers and proponents deny. Usually around the twenty-year mark enough evidence surfaces that a significant number of doctors begin to sound the alarm about safety. But historically, it is another ten years, for a total of 30 years on the market, before steps are taken to curtail over prescribing. By that time the manufacturers patents have expired, and they go on to the next latest, greatest drug.

At 16 years in the marketplace Prozac is nearing the 20-year mark, and with these new FDA warnings it looks like things are right on schedule. We can learn from history; we don't have to let these drugs continue to be over prescribed for 10 more years.

6
Antidepressants and Pain

Over the years antidepressants have evolved in treatment for depression and pain. Monoamine oxidase inhibitors (MAOs) were introduced in the 1950s and are still used today, a specific MAO-B inhibitor should be available in patch form soon. In the 1960s tricyclic antidepressants (TCAs) were introduced and the 1980s were known for the Selective Serotonin Reuptake Inhibitors (SSRIs). Over the past decade antidepressants have taken a new direction, they have been designed to regulate not only serotonin but norepinephrine as well; these dual action drugs are Effexor, Serzone, and Remeron. Next year a new Serotonin-Norepinephrine Reuptake Inhibitor (SNRI) will probably be available.

In 1998, Stephen Stahl theorized that the neurotransmitters; serotonin, dopamine, and norepinephrine affected mood. More specifically Stahl believed that serotonin and norepinephrine affected anxiety while dopamine regulated motivation, pleasure and reward.

Traditional treatment of patients with chronic pain usually will include antidepressants. Pain brings on depression further feeding the cycle of pain. Most physicians do not consider antidepressants to be addictive, but they are. You cannot just stop taking an antidepressant; dangerous side effects often accompany the *cold turkey* method. Tapering off slowly is the best way to stop taking an antidepressant.

Pain is an indication that something is wrong, but this

could be physical pain or psychosomatic pain. Physical pain may be from arthritis or a physical injury. Psychosomatic pain occurs as a result of mental stress such as a tension headache caused a conflict with your significant other. Usually the first reaction to pain is to reach for an over-the-counter (OTC) drug such as Motrin, Aleve, Advil, Naprosyn, aspirin, or prescription drugs like Feldene, Lodeine, Anaprox, Indocin, Celebrex, Vioxx, Voltaren, Bextra, etc. to relieve a headache or back pain. All of these are classified as NSAIDS (non-steroidal anti-inflammatory drugs) and have many dangerous side effects. The 3rd leading cause of death in the U.S. is drug side effects; over 6000 people die from NSAID use each year; in Western countries up to 70% of the population use analgesics on a regular basis for various kinds of pain. High level use of OTC analgesics often correlate with depression and the use of alcohol, caffeine, and nicotine. More than 4 grams of aspirin or acetaminophen a day, over a long period of time, indicates abuse.

Manipulation of mood changes perception and expression of pain. Clinical studies show tricyclic antidepressants (TCAs) enhance both serotonin and norepinephrine, and have been proven to decrease pain. While both SSRIs and tricyclics are effective for depression, the tricyclics are more effective for depression with pain, but the SSRIs are safer. The use of TCA antidepressants for chronic pain conditions such as fibromyalgia, post herpetic neuralgia (after shingles), and diabetic neuropathy respond to TCAs due to their dual action on serotonin and norepinephrine.

TCAs cause a myriad of side effects such as dry mouth, blurred vision, sexual dysfunction, weight gain, drowsiness, and dizziness. Over time TCAs often lose their effectiveness to relieve depression and pain. The loss of effectiveness results because the body has depleted its stores of neurotransmitters; tricyclics do not encourage the natural production of neurotransmitters so the body is not making enough. At this point physicians usually increase the dose of TCAs, but this increases risk of TCA side effects, increases risk for interactions with other medications, and further increases addiction.

Norepinephrine transmission comes from the locus ceruleus neurotransmitter system while serotonin is from the raphe nucleus system. Both regions of the brain influence the origins of depression and pain. Research suggests GABA may participate in the pain pathway as well. Chronic pain patients report a decrease in pain with the use of GABA modulators such as GABApentin, an antiepileptic drug. Elevations of Substance P exist in pain patients, but the exact role of the substance is still elusive. There are high concentrations of Substance P in the amygdala, this region is thought to be critical for the regulation of affective behavior and neurochemical responses to stress. Currently there are no known drugs targeting Substance P. Research shows that 30% of the population does not respond to any current drug therapies for depression.

Each individual has a unique biochemistry. Depression is a biochemical indication that not enough neurotransmitters are in production. Biochemical makeup may be responsible for deficiencies of particular neurotransmitters, such as serotonin. Low levels of serotonin are synonymous with depression, anxiety, aggression, mood swings, and feeling out of control. Low serotonin levels contribute to pain by lowering the pain threshold and increasing sensitivity to pain.

Drugs do not address biochemistry; they lose their effectiveness over time and can cause severe addiction. The use of amino acids such as 5-HTP elevates serotonin levels and puts back in the brain what naturally belongs there. This elevates mood while decreasing pain. Use the amino acids, Tyrosine and Phenylalanine, to elevate norepinephrine and dopamine levels. Mood Sync, a combination formula containing GABA, Tyrosine, and 5-HTP, restores the levels of three major neurotransmitters in the brain—GABA, norepinephrine, and serotonin.

The use of NSAIDs or COX2 inhibitors (Vioxx, Celebrex) for arthritis is standard medical practice. Essential fatty acids (EFAs) are natural anti-inflammatory agents and can be used in place of Vioxx or Celebrex. Using pure, distilled high quality EFAs will eliminate reflux and bad after taste. Another alternative is the herb Boswellia. Boswellia has been used for thousands of years and continues to be used in the East for arthritis; there has been great success in treating both rheumatoid and osteoarthritis.

Sleep disturbances are common for pain patients. Sleep is disrupted due to chronic pain and lack of sleep can occur from the same chronic pain, it's a vicious cycle. Standard treatment is to use antidepressants to positively affect both sleep and pain. Sometimes physicians add sleeping pills like Ambien or Sonata.

With the virtual pharmacy that exists in the brain, why become dependant on drugs and their many possible side effects?

7
Antidepressants and Breast Cancer

Experimental and epidemiologic studies suggest use of certain antidepressant medications may be associated with an increased risk of breast cancer. Women using some tricyclic antidepressants for longer than two-years had a twofold increase of breast cancer, while women who took the SSRI drug, Paxil, experienced a sevenfold increased risk. Dr. Michelle Cotterchio and colleagues from the division of Preventive Oncology, Cancer Care Ontario, Toronto, Canada, published these findings in the *American Journal of Epidemiology*, (May 15, 2000).

Smith Kline Beecham responded to Dr. Cotterchio's article in letters to the editor by saying the study was much too small and patients used in the study had been exposed to Prozac, another popular SSRI. Dr. Cotterchio defended her stance by saying future studies would be required to confirm these findings. However, animal studies support the hypothesis that antidepressants may be tumor promoters.

Following the article, during an interview, Dr. Cotterchio said the findings should be treated cautiously. "You can't say from a single observational study, what people should or shouldn't do." However, at the same time, Dr. Cotterchio said that, personally, she would consider switching from Paxil to another drug because the research showed the magnitude of risk.

Another study published in the *British Journal of Cancer*

(January 2002) demonstrated heavy exposure to certain tri-cyclic antidepressants was associated with an increased risk for breast cancer 11-15 years *after* exposure to the medication. Research shows not all tricyclics promote breast cancer. However, the TCAs, Asendin (amoxapine), Anafranil (clomipramine), Norpramin (desipramine), and Surmontil (trimipramine) showed a great increased risk of breast cancer in women. Laboratory experiments reveal these five drugs damage DNA, and observational studies prove the long-term effects on women by increased cases of breast cancer.

Many doctors seem hesitant to cause a stir when drugs start showing adverse reactions. They make statements such as "more research needs to be done," "women should not panic, and stop taking medication for depression." Since the advent of the SSRIs, more and more people are taking these drugs for a wide variety of problems. Besides depression, these drugs are commonly used to treat chronic pain, premenstrual syndrome (PMS), bulimia, attention deficit hyperactivity disorder, panic disorder, obsessive-compulsive behavior (OCD), and smoking cessation.

Neurotransmitters don't exist just in the brain. Only 5% of the body's total serotonin is in the brain, while 95% is found throughout the body. Serotonin plays a major role in controlling a number of hormones. According to Allan Steingart, assistant professor of psychiatry at the University of Toronto, SSRIs are endocrine disrupters, and they can alter estrogen levels. Since SSRIs manipulate serotonin and estrogen levels, are you at increased risk for breast cancer, if you take or have taken a SSRI?

The good news is you don't have to expose yourself to potentially dangerous drugs. Neurotransmitters are produced from amino acids. Research documents that when you supplement with the proper amino acids and nutrients, behavior disorders are corrected.

8
Orthomolecular Therapy

*O**rthomolecular therapy*** means supplying the cells with the right mixture of nutrients. Many diseases are known to be the result of the wrong balance of essential nutrients in the body. Adjusting the diet, eliminating junk foods and ingesting the proper doses of essential vitamins, minerals and amino acids, can correct the chemical imbalance of disease.

The orthomolecular approach helps patients become more aware of our dangerously polluted environment and nutrient-stripped refined foods. The orthomolecular approach is both corrective and preventative. Meganutrient therapy has become a part of orthomolecular medicine. While it is becoming widely recognized that orthomolecular therapy cures patients by correcting brain chemical imbalances, it is not widely known that in certain combinations, meganutrients can be as immediately effective as potent painkillers or tranquilizers. Meganutrients treat the whole person's biochemical imbalances; benefits can be seen immediately as well as long-term. The type of treatment offered by orthomolecular doctors and therapists varies, but the mainstream of work focuses upon meganutrient therapy and diagnostic tests, and treatment with adequate nutrients is a distinguishing characteristic of orthomolecular medicine.

Orthomolecular therapy considers every individual biochemically unique. Every patient has a very different nutrient and amino acid requirement; proper application of this therapy meets each individual's need. The mind and body are in a state of homeostasis–a condition where everything in the body is in balance and capable of resisting environmental changes, while regulating internal metabolic function.

Nutrition affects every tissue of the body. Under conditions of poor nutrition, the kidneys stop filtering, the stomach stops digesting, the adrenals stop secreting and other organs follow suit.

Good nutrition is essential to the preservation of health and the prevention of disease, and optimum intake of essential vitamins, minerals, and amino acids. Breakthroughs in nutritional science have given patients hope beyond drugs. The late Dr. Roger Williams at the University of Texas, Clayton Foundation opened new doors into the understanding of the brain's chemistry and the use of amino acids and nutrients. Dr. William's research demonstrated for maximum function the brain must be constantly fed. The brain is a 24-hour organ that *never* sleeps requiring continual nourishment. Yet, the brain is the most undernourished organ in the body. Proper nourishment utilizing proper amino acids and nutrients is the answer.

Meganutrient therapy has become a part of orthomolecular medicine. As the field continues to grow, we now recognize that all our biological interactions with food, water, air and light, *in the proper amounts, play an important role in good health and prevention of illness.* The sum total of orthomolecular therapy is *putting back in the body and brain what belongs there.*

9
Grief Reactions

At some point in your life, you will go through grief and bereavement. More than likely when you go through bereavement, your doctor will offer you tranquilizers or antidepressants to help you get through the tough time. If you take tranquilizers not only do you run a risk of dependence, but because drugs dull emotions, you will be unable to adjust to the loss or altered situation. Well-meaning physicians will offer you tranquilizers, anti-depressants, pain medication, or sleeping pills.

Grief is a debt we must all pay at some point in our life. Yes, it is a tough time, but a time that you learn to put your faith in the Lord and go on. If you use any psychiatric drugs, you are only postponing what you must face at some point. Do not be afraid to express your emotions. Grief is a way of saying good-bye, and "I miss you." Grief leaves many people dependent, and drugs become a crutch with all your feelings bottled up. You just have to face the grief again when the medication stops. You may feel severe guilt about not facing your loss, or not having been able to say good-bye, or not grieving at the *proper* time. In later years, suppressed emotions can come to the surface and cause withdrawal, depression, and delayed grief. As suppressed emotions release, old fears, phobias, guilt, and anxiety are resolved, and you regain your self-respect. Then, you can finally face old conflicts, traumas, and unresolved anxieties.

During the grieving process, if you cared for a sick relative, you are hit harder and longer by grief and depression. A study sponsored by the National Institute of Mental Health found 30% of caregivers suffered from clinical depression or anxiety, while their loved one was alive. Four years later, 25% still suffer symptoms while 10% of non-care giving relatives were depressed for four years after the death.

Nutritional support is very important for caregivers. The prolonged intense stress and grief depletes their neurotransmitters, and they must be replenished. Grief is a major transition period in our lives. Your pain and grief will not go away if you are using drugs or alcohol. Find a therapist with empathetic understanding. Express your feelings and fears, and allow the healing process to begin. Take one day at a time, and feed your brain nutrients daily.

10
Amino Acids and Nutrients

Amino acid supplements have a positive effect on people suffering from addictions, whether the addiction is to alcohol, cocaine, marijuana, or prescribed medications for anxiety, pain, or depression. The use of any of these psychoactive substances alters and depletes the brain of naturally occurring neuro-nutrients and neurotransmitters that allow us to think, make decisions and enjoy life. Restoring the balance of amino acids in the brain and body assists in handling the stress of withdrawal and provides the brain with the correct nutrients for normalization of function.

At the Pain & Stress Center we have been using amino acids and other nutrients successfully to treat anxiety, depression, Attention Deficit Disorder, and chronic pain for over 20 years. The use of nutrition to treat these disorders is grounded in solid science beginning with Linus Pauling, Nobel Prize laureate in 1954. Pauling coined the word, *orthomolecular,* to describe the process of "establishing the right molecules in the brain by varying the concentrations of substances normally present and required for optimum health." This research has been built upon by doctors such as Carl Pfeiffer, Ph.D., M.D., author of *Nutrition and Mental Illness*, and Eric Braverman, M.D., in his book *The Healing Nutrients Within*, and Candace Pert, Ph.D., author of *Molecules of Emotion.* Candace Pert discovered the opiate receptor and gave us a much broader understanding of GABA and how neurotransmitters function throughout the brain and body.

The philosophy of putting back in the brain what belongs there has been documented as very effective in the treatment of psychiatric disorders, and is the only solution when trying to come off prescribed medications, or overcome addiction to any substance. Medications, drugs, and alcohol affect us because they work on our own naturally occurring brain chemicals—the neurotransmitters. Medications alter neurotransmitter functioning by decreasing receptor sites and reducing receptor site sensitivity. When medication is withdrawn quickly, the brain is unable to function normally because of the drug-induced changes. People often continue to take medications for years—simply because they fear the symptoms of withdrawal. Fear is the strongest emotion we experience. If you provide the brain with the proper amino acids and nutrients in the amount needed, withdrawal is not an agonizing or impossible task.

A forty-one year old teacher treated at the Pain & Stress Center had been on Paxil for three years. He had been prescribed the medication for a situational depression that had resolved. He was ready to discontinue treatment. When prescribing Paxil his doctor had not indicated that this drug would be difficult to stop. The patient was very surprised when he stopped taking the medication. Within two days, he was unable to function due to *severe* withdrawal symptoms. Thinking these symptoms must be a fluke, he tried to stop Paxil several times. Each time he always experienced the same debilitating symptoms of electrical shocks, vertigo and mind-numbing depression. When he contacted the Pain & Stress Center, we made recommendations for a supplementation program as well as advised him on a reduction schedule. Two months later, he called our office to say he had been off Paxil for two weeks. By following his nutritional program, his withdrawal was easy. He continued with the supplementation program, we designed for him. He reported feeling the best he had ever felt. The key to his success was taking specific doses of amino acids daily to balance the brain chemistry.

Amino acids are the building blocks of proteins in the body. If you were to take all the water and fat out of the body, 75% of the remainder would be proteins. These primary amino acids join together in different combinations to form our muscles, cell membranes, enzymes, and neurotransmitters. Neurotransmitters, the biochemical components of thought and emotions, are produced in the brain. Increasing dietary intake of amino acids affects the concentration of those neurotransmitters from which they metabolically derive. Abram Hoffer, M.D. states in *Putting It All Together*, "Your nutritional status is as good as the last meal eaten." So, the neurotransmitters, dopamine, norepinephrine, serotonin, histamine, GABA, and endorphins can increase or decrease depending upon excesses or deficiencies in their parent amino acids. Because medications deplete these neurotransmitters, it is vitally important to provide the brain with adequate raw materials to restore levels for healthy functioning. We are all biochemically unique and no two people require the same amounts of amino acids. Each individual's distinct chemical composition and brain function are unique to their lifestyle and nutrient intake.

Neurons come from neurotransmitters via amino acids. Millions of times a second, signals fire within the brain in a *Star Wars* fashion, involving mental, emotional, and physical events. Neurotransmitter synthesis occurs within the neuron from precursors delivered to the cell from the outside. Each second this process endlessly repeats, so the demand for brain nourishment is great.

GABA

Probably the least understood part of the entire limbic system is the ring of cerebral cortex called the limbic cortex. This part functions as a crossover zone where signals are transmitted from the rest of the cortex into the limbic system. The function of the limbic cortex appears to be a link to the cerebral cortex for the control of behavior. Anxiety occurs when the limbic system—the part of the brain that stores anxiety messages—begins to release numerous signals, and simultaneously, a physiological response starts to take place—the fight-or-flight syndrome. To an anxious person, this threatens a potential loss of control.

The unceasing alert signals from the limbic system eventually overwhelm the cortex. Then the ability of the cortex and the rest of the stress network to accommodate the crisis become exhausted. The balance between the limbic system and the cortex goes to pieces, often leading people into erratic or irrational fear—or making them want to reach for their favorite substance.

The ability of the cortex to communicate with the limbic system and the rest of the brain in an orderly fashion depends critically on inhibition, namely GABA (Gamma Amino Butyric Acid). GABA inhibits the cells from firing, diminishing the excitatory messages reaching the frontal cortex. GABA seems to lower the excitatory level of the cell that is about to receive the incoming information. If the anxiety, stress, or fear continues, GABA's ability to block the messages is decreased, and finally the process by which the signals are rated for priority breaks down, the frontal cortex is literally bombarded with anxiety messages. A full-blown panic attack follows.

With the limbic system firing broadside fight-or-flight signals at the frontal cortex, the subject's ability to reason is diminished. The effects now can include fear of dying, pounding heart, sweating, trembling, tightness, weakness, loss of control, disorientation—the list is endless. Research has shown GABA can actually mimic the tranquilizing effect of Valium and Librium but without the heavy sedation effect of these drugs. Sandy Shaw and Durk Pearson first released this information for publication in 1982 in *Life Extension Magazine*. Since that time, numerous published studies show the successful use of GABA with anxiety-prone individuals and phobics. Many addicts, both drug and alcohol, have a tremendous problem with anxiety and anticipatory fear.

Research reports have shown that a person, who constantly experiences *what-if* type anxiety, or *anticipatory* fear, has empty GABA receptors in the brain. The brain can be bombarded with random firings of excitatory messages. GABA receptor sites in the brain prevent the reception of all the random firings so that the brain does not become overwhelmed. In *Lancet*, August 14, 1982, a research report about tranquilizers and GABA transmission clearly stated that GABA is a major inhibitory transmitter in the mammalian central nervous system. The agents that raise the brain's GABA concentration possess a sedative anticonvulsant property.

After publication of information about GABA, the public quickly became aware of the potentiality of GABA as an anti-anxiety formula. A survey of the medical journals shows over 300 articles (case studies, clinical reports, etc.) on GABA by orthomolecular psychiatrists and researchers.

GABA and the neurons that utilize it as an inhibitory neurotransmitter are found throughout the central nervous system. In view of the growing knowledge regarding the regulation of the physiology of the central nervous system, GABA is assuming an ever-enlarging role as a major influence on drugs, in many cases replacing them (for example, Valium and Xanax). Preliminary pharmacological and clinical data have already demonstrated the usefulness of GABA in exploring human disease.

As of 2004, clinical work at the Pain & Stress Center in San Antonio using pure GABA 750 mg, demonstrated the effectiveness of GABA as a muscle relaxant as well as an anti-anxiety agent. Pure GABA is tasteless, odorless, and colorless; it readily dissolves in water. In 100 patients followed at the Pain & Stress Center, GABA 750 reduced the level of tension in the muscles in 7 to 10 minutes. GABA is helpful in reducing anxiety. There are GABA receptor sites throughout the body as well as the brain.

Dr. K. J. Berman at Mt. Sinai School of Medicine published an extensive review in *Clinical Neuropharmacology* (1985) entitled "Progabide: A New GABA Mimetric Electric Agent in Clinical Use." Dr. Berman sums up the research and results of the clinical chemistry, the role of GABA, and the influences in the central nervous system. In 1985, the most valid research published on GABA relates to anxiety. In 2004, GABA's benefits are still being expanded. GABA not only aids anxiety sufferers, but also lessens muscle tension, and aids Parkinson's symptoms, as well as inhibiting the desire for alcohol and cocaine. Soon this extremely versatile amino acid will make more major contributions to aid those suffering from pain, stress, anxiety, and addiction. For further information, read my book, *GABA, The Anxiety Amino Acid*.

Glutamine, The Surprising Brain Fuel

Glutamine is the third most abundant amino acid in the blood and brain. Glutamine provides a major alternative fuel source for the brain when blood sugar levels are low.

Glutamine, an inhibitory neurotransmitter, functions as a precursor for GABA, the anti-anxiety amino acid. Glutamine helps the brain dispose of waste ammonia, a protein breakdown by-product that irritates brain cells even at low levels. Recent scientific research regarding glutamine demonstrates its link to the most important functions of the body's vital organs and musculoskeletal system. Glutamine aids the body in muscle development when illness causes muscle wasting that can occur following a high fever, chronic stress, illness or a traumatic accident.

Glutamine plays an important role in the functioning of the immune system. Glutamine helps with the multiplication of selected white cells, which strengthen the body's defense system. Glutamine aids other immune cells in killing bacteria. Glutamine aids in healing wounds, supports pancreatic growth, and maintains and supports glutathione, an important antioxidant.

Scientists at National Institute of Health (NIH) in 1970 found glutamine, not glucose, is the most important nutrient for the intestinal tract. During times of illness, the body uses more glutamine to aid tissue repair in the kidneys, intestines, and liver. For many years, glutamine was considered a nonessential amino acid, but research the past several years has brought forth a wave of new important information to change this view. Every day more research is being conducted on the healing power of amino acids. Glutamine, along with GABA and glycine, are rapidly becoming the most important therapeutic amino acids of the twenty-second century.

Neurotransmitters are vital to brain function. The amino acid trio of glutamine, GABA, glycine with B6, a cofactor, provides the major inhibitory neurotransmitters in the brain. Glutamine is found in the nerves of the hippocampus, the memory center of the brain; in the cranial nerves; and in many other areas of the brain. B6 must be supplemented along with amino acids to enable their metabolism. GABA and glutamine *are not only* found in the brain, but in receptor cites *throughout the body*. Amino acids can and do change mind, mood, memory and behavior.

If you crave alcohol, Dr. Roger Williams, pioneer in glutamine research, found that 3,000 to 4,000 milligrams of glutamine daily will stop the craving for alcohol and decrease the craving for sweets. Since glutamine is tasteless and mixes with water or any liquid, it is easy to take. Our patients also reported a lift from mental and physical fatigue. One alcoholic stopped drinking when glutamine was administered daily. Two years later the patient was still alcohol free, without the craving for alcohol. He maintained a nutritional support program that addressed his brain deficiencies.

Dr. Lorene Rogers, researcher at the University of Texas, Clayton Foundation, reported several cases in which glutamine was successful over placebo in treating alcohol cravings. Glutamine was given to one group of alcoholics and placebos to the other. The group taking at least three thousand milligrams of glutamine daily was free of alcohol craving.

Glutamine is converted to energy by the brain; it is

the brain's major source of fuel. Glutamine is converted to GABA with the help of magnesium. Without continued high energy in the brain, the rest of the mind and body will NOT function correctly. The brain requires a huge supply of glucose and oxygen to perform properly. This energy supply is delivered via the bloodstream. Proper circulation ensures the brain will have the energy it needs.

Glutamine is the main nutrient needed for intestinal repair. Glutamine has proven beneficial in cases of leaky gut syndrome that is being seen more often today due to the increased use of anti-inflammatory medications such as Motrin, Advil, Ibuprofen, Dolobid, Anaprox, Aleve, Naprosyn, Celebrex, Vioxx, aspirin, etc.

Unfortunately, foods are not a good source of glutamine. The foods highest in glutamine include meat, chicken and eggs, but in the raw form. Cooking or heat inactivates glutamine, so your best source is in supplement form.

Glutamine, truly an amazing amino acid, provides multiple benefits. With continued research, other important factors will be found that will improve our quality of life. Glutamine is available in capsule and powder forms.

Phenylalanine

Phenylalanine, an essential amino acid, is necessary for life. Phenylalanine converts to tyrosine in the liver. Tyrosine then forms the neurotransmitters dopamine, norepinephrine and epinephrine, members of the catecholamines family. The formation of these neurotransmitters is affected by diet, by making more or less of the respective precursors available to the brain you can increase or decrease the levels of those neurotransmitters.

The rate that each of these is synthesized is affected by the availability of the particular substance. The amount of dopamine, norepinephrine, and epinephrine that is available to the brain is predisposed by the amount of amino acid precursors provided.

Phenylalanine Pathway

Phenylalanine → Tyrosine → Dopamine → Norepinephrine → Epinephrine

L-phenylalanine is the raw substance that produces several compounds of the catecholamines family. Catecholamines are responsible for the transmission of nerve impulses. A good supply of phenylalanine (or tyrosine) must be present in the blood so the adrenal medulla and the nerve cells can rapidly produce these catecholamines. All of the amino acids are the building blocks of protein, but phenylalanine is one of the few amino acids readily converted into brain compounds that control a person's moods.

The body requires phenylalanine to rebuild proteins; its most important role may be in the production of the critical neurotransmitters and hormones—epinephrine (adrenaline), dopa, norepinephrine, dopamine, thyroxine, and tri-iodthyronine. Phenylalanine is found in a variety of foods in small amounts. Inadequate amounts of phenylalanine lead to low levels of norepinephrine that can result in severe depression. These neurotransmitters control the whole basic process of nerve impulse transmission. Epinephrine is important because it is excreted at the nerve terminals in the hypothalamus. Norepinephrine is excreted at the sympathetic nerve endings giving a basic fight-or-flight response. Thus, norepinephrine affects the immediate postsynaptic cells.

Norepinephrine, the principal neurotransmitter at the peripheral nerve endings of the sympathetic nervous system, is the neurotransmitter in certain central synapses, and is stored in the presynaptic vesicles. Whenever the body endures a tremendous amount of stress, it places an enormous load on the adrenal glands; many times, the epinephrine and norepinephrine levels—especially the norepinephrine levels—become either very low or depleted. Low levels of norepinephrine can cause depression, and stress can cause pain, depression, anxiety, uncertainty, and fear.

A depressed person may become more depressed when he is alone or in a particular situation which gives rise to distraction. With no happiness in his life, he feels hopeless and helpless about the future. Without energy or interest, often he or she will reach for a drink or drug.

Depression exhibits many faces. Depression constitutes a wide spectrum from sadness or the "blues" that everyone experiences at one time or another to reactive depression caused by the loss of someone or something loved. It extends to psychotic depression in which contact with reality is lost, and there may even be thoughts of suicide or—the ultimate loss—the actual act of suicide. Psychotic depression may or may not be endogenous (i.e., self-produced) depression. It can actually be diet induced. Depression is one of the most common disorders of the mind. Often it is treated with antidepressants and/or tranquilizers.

The affective disorders are divided into two types: unipolar and bipolar. Unipolar is characterized by depression or mania alone. Bipolar is depicted by both depression and mania. The difference is important, for the origin is probably different; likewise, the two disorders have different pharmacological responses.

The widely accepted hypothesis for affective disorders is the catecholamine hypothesis. Although it has various forms, the simplest concept is depression is caused by faulty metabolism. To support the theory more evidence is available for depression than mania.

Traditional medicine treats depression with a number of medications. Two types of drugs affect the norepinephrine levels. Monoamine oxidase inhibitors (MAOs) inhibit the breakdown of norepinephrine. Tricyclic antidepressants prevent the reuptake of norepinephrine, and dopamine from the synaptic cleft. Still another medication used in the treatment of depression is the psychostimulants, such as amphetamine and methylphenidate. These drugs work by increasing the amount of norepinephrine available at the synaptic cleft. The extra norepinephrine is available due to an increased release from the storage vesicles, inhibiting monoamine reuptake. To date, a single mechanism does not fit all the facts of the affective disorders and their pharmacological and therapeutic responses. The cause of depression does not appear to be a single entity.

L-phenylalanine has been used to increase the level of norepinephrine in the brain. The neurotransmitters, especially norepinephrine, are responsible for an elevation and positive moods, alertness and ambition in a person.

Sometimes drugs such as antidepressants artificially elevate the norepinephrine level; these drugs work by blocking the norepinephrine from reentering the pouches within the neuron. This blocking causes an artificial manipulation of norepinephrine that leads to an elevation of mood. In actuality, this aggravates the original problem. The natural way to normalize the brain and nerve level of norepinephrine is by providing adequate levels of the amino acids L-phenylalanine or L-tyrosine.

DLPA—Depression and Pain

Most people think of their emotions as separate from their bodies and unconnected with the chemistry of their brain cells; however, depression, irritability, and anxiety all reflect the functioning of the brain. When certain nutrients are not supplied to the brain, we experience an array of negative emotions, tending to lose our coping abilities in response to stressful circumstances we confront each day of our lives.

Although the brain equals only 2% of our total body weight, 25% of our metabolic activity takes place there. This is probably the reason why the brain is so sensitive to nutritional deficiency. Nutrients can cause important changes in the chemical composition of substances in the brain, with corresponding changes in our feelings. Scientific studies show that taking particular amino acids alleviates mental depression, apathy, peevishness, and the desire to be left alone.

About one in five Americans has significant symptoms of depression, more than 2.5 million are being treated for it, and about 50 million can expect to suffer from it at some point in their lives. Classic, full-blown depression has been described as "the loss of the capacity to enjoy life combined with decreased thought and movement." Depression can appear as grief, but may manifest itself through a series of emotional states so extreme that the outcome is suicide or total withdrawal.

Of course, a preoccupation with death or suicide is an obvious symptom, but often depression is not obvious because the person does not feel *sad*. These *masked depression* symptoms involve changes in sleeping patterns, such as insomnia, early morning waking, constant sleepiness, or changes in eating patterns—either overeating or loss of appetite. The person may be anxious or have excessive complaints about body functions and chronic pain, especially headaches, but also indigestion or constipation. Both hair and skin may feel dry and lack luster, while blood pressure has a tendency to be high. He or she experiences an inability to enjoy customary pleasures and a concomitant loss of sex drive, loss of energy, extreme fatigue, difficulty concentrating and making decisions, irritability, and possibly temperamental outbursts.

Endogenous depression exhibits symptoms of guilt, self-hate, feelings of worthlessness, apathy, crying spells, and a desire to be left alone. Women are more susceptible to depression than men—1 woman in 6, compared to 1 man in 12. Some think women there may be some connection to the female reproductive hormone cycles. In addition, some diseases, such as hypothyroidism (under active thyroid gland), can produce depression, while others, such as arthritis or heart disease, commonly bring on a depressive reaction. Overall, depression can be a result of nutritional deficiency that puts further stress on the body. Without the proper nutritional attention, depression has a very deleterious effect on the general health.

Treatment

DLPA (or DL-phenylalanine) is effective in the treatment of depression. Since 1974, studies demonstrate DLPA to be particularly beneficial in cases of endogenous depression. Endogenous depression is characterized by a decrease in energy and interest, feelings of worthlessness, and a pervasive sense of helplessness to control the course of one's life. Significant improvement has also been achieved using DLPA in people suffering from reactive depression (thought to be caused by environmental influences such as a death in the family) and involutional depression (an aging-related depression). DLPA has also shown itself to be effective for other types of depression, including the depressive phase of manic-depression, schizophrenic depression, and post-amphetamine depression.

Phenylalanine is one of the *essential* amino acids, and it must be obtained through the diet. The type of phenylalanine our bodies require is L-phenylalanine, while the type found to be most effective against depression is D-phenylalanine. D-phenylalanine mirrors L-phenylalanine in its molecular structure. DLPA or the DL-form is the preferable form for depression and pain. DLPA is a 50/50 mixture of D-phenylalanine and L-phenylalanine. They do not interact but follow separate transport and metabolic pathways. In other words, 750 mg of DLPA behaves like 375 mg of pure D–phenylalanine plus 375 mg of L-phenylalanine.

At this time, it appears that DLPA has three separate antidepressant effects in the body: it increases production of PEA (phenylethylamine), endorphins, and norepinephrine. These biochemical changes are not isolated but rather create a synergistic overlap that accounts for the terrific result of DLPA in the treatment of depression.

Although D-phenylalanine is very rare in nature, all mammals, including man, are able to metabolize it. Part of the metabolic process involves conversion to phenylethylamine or PEA. PEA is a neurotransmitter-type substance that bears a close structural resemblance to the stimulant drug amphetamine. It seems to be a natural stimulant. This characteristic prompted mental health researchers to speculate that a deficiency of PEA in the nervous system might be a cause of depression. This concept gained support when research demonstrated that depressed patients were not just low in PEA, they were "immeasurably low."

In a series of studies in the late 70s, it was also found that every major treatment for depression indirectly elevated levels of PEA in the brain. Both D– and L–forms of phenylalanine are directly converted to PEA. However, D–phenylalanine has been reported to induce greater, more prolonged increases than L-phenylalanine alone. A second way DLPA may act as an antidepressant is in its ability to inhibit enzymes that break down endorphins and enkephlins. Endorphins are the body's own morphine-like substances whose presence may account for the euphoria experienced by runners, joggers, and other enthusiasts of aerobic exercise. Endorphin concentration in the brain may be critical in mood regulation and pain. If a sufficient number of the receptors in the brain are filled with endorphins and enkephalins, a person feels a sense of well-being and reduced pain. However, if for some reason the endorphin level reduces and too few receptors are filled, the deficiency causes a person to feel a sense of urgency and irritation. In a similar way, if the production is too high and an excessive number of receptors are filled, a person feels a sense of euphoria that is usually followed by a letdown. This is natural, and is a major cause of the *ups and downs* everyone experiences in life.

If drugs such as heroin or morphine are consumed, these drugs take the place of endorphins and enkephalins at the receptors and, if taken in quantity, activate a large number of receptors, creating an unnatural euphoria. A person feels great for a while, but the drug has a serious side effect. It causes the body to shut down the production of natural endorphins and enkephalins. Then, as the drug wears off, the feeling of need becomes greater than ever.

If drug consumption continues over a period of time, the ability of the body to produce endorphins and enkephalins is reduced, and the person becomes dependent on the drug.

A patient who has been taking narcotics or drugs for a while has desensitized his endorphin receptors. Even if he desired to quit using the narcotics, his body would not respond to an endorphin release. He must gradually reduce his intake of drugs to slowly reactivate his endorphin receptor sites.

In fact, clinical research has shown that endorphins administered intravenously can trigger sudden, dramatic antidepressant actions, even in suicidal patients. Essentially, DLPA works because it inhibits endorphin-degrading enzymes so that the endorphins produced by the brain last longer.

Alcohol has been found to cause the production of chemicals called tetrahydroisoquinolines, or TIQs, which have effects similar to morphine or heroin. They fill the enkephalin receptors, produce an unnatural euphoria, and reduce the output of the natural endorphins and enkephalins. The long-term use of large amounts of alcohol produces a permanent urgent need for alcohol, and the craving for more alcohol or another drink.

DLPA can be converted to the brain neurotransmitter, norepinephrine. A deficiency of norepinephrine was the first brain chemical deficiency believed to be involved in severe depression. Like PEA, norepinephrine is a natural stimulant. Both D- and L- phenylalanine serve as its precursors, although they follow somewhat different metabolic pathways. Most antidepressant drugs are designed to increase the amount of norepinephrine in the central nervous system, but by very different means than DLPA.

Antidepressant drugs, such as tricyclics, can be effective

in reducing symptoms of depression. Unfortunately, this is where their usefulness ends. They can cause numerous adverse side effects such as seizures, drowsiness, nausea, and anorexia. Tricyclic antidepressants can stimulate neurotransmitter release for mood elevation, but they prevent reabsorption of neurotransmitters into nerve terminals. This depletes our cellular stores of neurotransmitter material and interferes with proper brain function. DLPA can serve to restore brain levels to normal.

In a recent double-blind controlled study, DLPA was found to be equally as effective as the tricyclic drug, Imipramine.

- DL-phenylalanine and Imipramine were given to depressed patients in equal dosages (150-200 mg/day) with 20 patients in each group.
- Psychopathological, neurologic, and somatic indices showed no differences between the two treatments.
- Automatic side effects "tended to be higher for the Imipramine patients."
- Antidepressant efficacy of DL-phenylalanine "seems to equal that of the tricyclic antidepressant, Imipramine."

Evidence indicates that DLPA may be useful in alleviating the mood disorders associated with PMS (premenstrual syndrome). Reports from clinical investigations have revealed that over 80% of all patients suffering from PMS have experienced good to complete relief by supplementing with DLPA.

DLPA dosage comes in capsules of 375 to 750 mg. The dosage is generally 4 to 8 capsules per day. Each capsule should be taken 30 minutes prior to meals. It is important that the capsules be taken in divided dosages throughout the day to get the antidepressant effect. Dosage can be varied with improvement, but must be individualized. People who suffer from PKU (phenylketonuria) should not use DLPA.

Key Factors of DLPA

1) DLPA is a highly safe, nontoxic substance when used in short-or long-term therapy.

2) DLPA does not induce excessive excitation or arousal in normal or depressed subjects.

3) Toxic overdose is impossible and there is generally a lack of potential for abuse.

4) DLPA does not cause adverse side effects.

Endogenous depression, which was discussed earlier in relation to DLPA, is a particularly insidious mental state. The person involved feels so worthless that they are unable to take action towards feeling better. When a person is depressed, they do not feel like taking good care of themselves. Of course, that is the very time a person needs to eat properly, get enough sleep, exercise regularly and take amino acids.

L-Tyrosine

Clinical findings indicate the amino acid L-tyrosine is helpful in overcoming depression, improving memory, and increasing mental alertness. Research has linked L-tyrosine deficiency to the development of depression in some oral contraceptive users.

Tyrosine is considered a nonessential amino acid because the body can make it from phenylalanine. Supplementing tyrosine can have a sparing effect on phenylalanine.

The body needs L-tyrosine to build many complex structural proteins and enzymes as well as neurotransmitters. The specific neurotransmitters derived from tyrosine are known collectively as the catecholamines; individually they are dopamine, norepinephrine and adrenaline.

These neurotransmitters are responsible for elevated and positive mood, alertness, and ambition. Medical researchers in the past have relied on increasing the brain and nerve levels of norepinephrine by using drugs, such as phenylpropanolamine and amphetamines that cause the release of norepinephrine, or block its return to storage, or slowing the destruction of L-tyrosine. However, such artificial manipulation often leads to depletion of neurotransmitter stores and the aggravation of the original problem. The natural solution is to normalize brain and nerve levels of norepinephrine by providing adequate levels of L-tyrosine.

Clinical studies have shown that L-tyrosine controls medication-resistant depression. Two studies published in 1980 are of interest. Dr. Alan J. Gelenberg of the Department of Psychiatry at Harvard Medical School published the first in the *American Journal of Psychiatry*. Dr. Gelenberg discussed the role of L-tyrosine in controlling anxiety and depression. He postulated that a lack of available L-tyrosine results in a deficiency of the hormone norepinephrine at a specific brain location, which, in turn, relates to mood problems such as depression.

Dr. Gelenberg treated patients having long-standing depression not responding to standard therapy by

Do Not Take Phenylalanine, Tyrosine Or DLPA With the Following Medications:

Caution: These Drugs Are Addictive.

Brand Name/ Generic Name	Half-life	Toxic Side Effect(s)
Tofranil (Imipramine)	11–15 hrs.	Sedation, weight gain, dizziness
Pamelor, Aventyl (Nortriptyline)	18–44 hrs.	Zonked feeling, mental dysfunction, lethargy, fatigue, mental dullness, sedation
Elavil (Amitriptyline)	31–46 hrs.	Dry mouth, constipation, blurred vision
Norpramin (Desipramine)	12–24 hrs.	Shakiness, problems sleeping, blurred vision
Sinequan (Doxepin)	8–24 hrs.	Constipation, nervousness, restlessness
Vivactil (Protriptyline)	67–89 hrs.	Confusion, weakness, irregular heartbeat
Wellbutrin (Bupropion)	8–24 hrs.	Agitation, anxiety, confusion
Desyrel (Trazodone)	3–9 hrs.	Blurred vision, fatigue, anger
Effexor (Venlafaxine)	16 hrs.	Insomnia, dry mouth, anxiety

These drugs must be used with caution. Once you begin using them you should not discontinue use abruptly. Consult a health care professional for assistance.

administering dietary supplements of L-tyrosine. Within two weeks of daily intakes of 1,000 milligrams per day of a Tyrosine supplement, tremendous improvement was noted. Patients were able to discontinue or reduce amphetamines to minimal levels in a matter of weeks.

Dr. I. Goldberg published the second study in *Lancet*. Allergy sufferers have also responded well to L-tyrosine supplementation, as well as those on weight loss programs.

Pearson reports that L-tyrosine supplementation is a preferred way to control appetite, rather than phenylpropanolamine or amphetamine administration, which causes norepinephrine release only.

Cocaine addiction has been helped with daily supplementation of doses of at least 3000 mg per day in divided dosages. Additionally, GABA in doses of 3000 mg per day has reduced the stress and anxiety associated with cocaine addiction. Other important amino acids and nutrients include DLPA—2000 mg per day, and glutamine 2000 mg per day.

5-HTP (5-Hydroxytryptophan)

Finally, there is help if you suffer from depression, sleep disorders, hyperactivity, chronic stress syndrome, PMS, obsessive/compulsive behavior, addiction, and carbohydrate craving. 5-HTP or 5-Hydroxytryptophan, a natural extract from the Griffonia plant seed, readily converts to serotonin in the brain.

Serotonin is a major neurotransmitter that is responsible for communication between nerve cells. Without neurotransmitters you would not be able to think, function or even live. Serotonin is released and received throughout the brain and spinal cord.

5-HTP is safe and effective. It is free from side effects and has no reported toxicity or contraindications. Researchers have observed a definite link between depression, addiction, obsessive/compulsive behavior and serotonin deficiency. Serotonin is the key to numerous brain functions; as the level decreases maladaptive behavior increases. The serotonin system is the largest single neurotransmitter system in the brain, influencing multiple functions such as moods, movement, behavior, and eating patterns. 5-HTP from the Griffonia seed has been established as a true solution to those who need more serotonin.

Tryptophan → 5-HTP → Serotonin

In the body, the amino acid, tryptophan, is converted to 5-HTP, which is then converted to serotonin. Serotonin undergoes additional conversions in the pineal gland to yield melatonin that is responsible for inducing sleep. Serotonin is the brain's master impulse controller for all emotions and drives. When your serotonin level is low, aggression and anger are often the first symptoms. Addictive and compulsive behavior, headaches, pain, and depression are also warning signals your brain is asking for more serotonin. Decreased serotonin levels in the brain are also associated with obesity and alcoholism; low serotonin causes the brain to send signals of hunger or craving

Millions of people have turned to SSRIs (Selective Serotonin Reuptake Inhibitors) to treat depression; drugs such as Prozac, Paxil, Zoloft, Luvox, Serzone, Celexa, Lexapro, and Effexor work by selective enhancement of serotonin levels. SSRIs prevent the presynaptic nerve from reabsorbing serotonin previously secreted. By inhibiting the normal process of reuptake these drugs cause an increase in brain serotonin levels. However they do not actually increase the production of neurotransmitters, so ultimately they create a serotonin deficiency. SSRIs can cause the brain to rev up. This can cause a false euphoria; mood swings as well as aggressive behavior.

5-HTP elevates the serotonin level of the brain naturally without side effects or drug dependency. Those using antidepressants for recovery from addiction or depression will not feel any relief for at least a month; the benefits of

5-HTP are felt within 24 to 48 hours. Michael J. Norden, M.D. in his best selling book, *Beyond Prozac,* described a patient who suffered from chronic anxiety and depression for most of her forty-four years. Prescription medication did not give her any relief so Dr. Norden decided to give her 5-HTP. She showed a marked improvement—both her anxiety and depression decreased remarkably. Dr. Norden found a 1993 study of patients with painful fibromyalgia showed a significant improvement using 5-HTP daily. Patients treated at the Pain & Stress Center with fibromyalgia, chronic pain syndrome, and headaches responded to treatment once 5-HTP was added to their daily program.

Low serotonin influences pain and headaches in different ways. Serotonin regulates blood flow to muscles; when levels are low from chronic stress syndrome, your muscles constantly contract. Muscles will stay in a contracted state causing an increase of muscle tension and pain. Pain is directly related to low serotonin.

5-HTP is synergistic with other supplements that enhance neurotransmitters such as GABA, glutamine, tyrosine, DLPA, and glycine. Magnesium prolongs the benefits of 5-HTP, especially magnesium chloride found in Mag Link. Chronic stress syndrome will deplete available serotonin as well as interfere with serotonin's ability to control behavior. Research has demonstrated a low serotonin level can change brain function, and impair learning. Most children and adults with A.D.D. and A.D.H.D. have low serotonin levels and a definite deficiency of needed neurotransmitters. Adding 5-HTP in the proper amounts can correct the imbalance. Scientists now believe low serotonin may be responsible for an increase in depression and drug use among teens and children. Teens with low serotonin levels are more prone to try recreational drugs

Serotonin Pathways

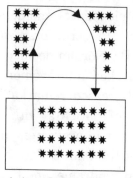 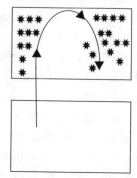

Serotonin is made from the amino acid, tryptophan or 5-HTP. Serotonin releases in the brain, and should recirculate so it can be utilized again.

Serotonin is blocked in the brain by SSRIs, antidepressants, and tricyclics. A person is at risk to develop Serotonin Syndrome.

or even prescription drugs to try to find relief. Low serotonin levels in the brain impair their ability to focus and reason. 5-HTP shows a lot of promise as a natural answer to a multitude of problems that plague adults and children. Given all of the information and scientific research, 5-HTP can have a profound effect on your quality of life.

5-HTP can be found individually or in combination formulas such as Mood Sync. Consider your particular problem and select the formula that best addresses your problem. Caution must be taken with children. Doses should be adjusted according to age, weight, and the particular problem. If you are using any prescription medications, be extremely cautious about taking 5-HTP. The two in combination could cause problems such as *serotonin syndrome*. Serotonin syndrome is a condition that causes symptoms of irrational euphoria, diarrhea, agitation, confusion, and gastrointestinal upset. Unfortunately, there is no treatment for Serotonin Syndrome except time. If you are taking SSRIs, you should not combine it with 5-HTP unless you decrease the amount of medication you are taking. If you are decreasing your medication, it is best to work with your doctor or health practitioner.

Special Note for Prozac Users

In *Vitamin Research News* March 1998, Dr. Ward Dean was asked if you could use 5-HTP with Prozac. According to Dr. Dean, "Yes, you can (and probably should) use 5-HTP with Prozac. However, you will probably have to reduce your dosage of Prozac after starting 5-HTP in order to prevent *serotonin excess syndrome.*

"SSRIs increase the amount of serotonin in the synaptic clefts between nerve endings, but they don't do anything to replace the tryptophan that is required for the body to manufacture serotonin. Consequently, we believe that many Prozac users become deficient in tryptophan, resulting in increased requirements for Prozac, which just makes the situation worse. Many former users of Prozac were able to completely discontinue their antidepressants by replacing them with 5-HTP (but only do this under guidance from a physician or qualified health care professional)."

Remember we are all biochemically individual; some people won't tolerate a low dose of 5-HTP while others require a larger dose. It is always advisable to start with a lower dose and increase to find the correct amount.

L-Theanine

L-theanine (L-T) is a free form amino acid found in green tea leaves. A relative newcomer to the supplement industry theanine is quickly being recognized as an important player in brain function. Theanine appears to have a role in the formation of the major inhibitory neurotransmitter, Gamma Amino Butyric Acid (GABA). GABA is the brains stop switch, without ample GABA, excitatory messages overwhelm the brain leading to anxiety and panic.

A study published in the *Journal of Food Science & Technology* in 1999 confirms theanine has a significant effect on the release of the neurotransmitters, dopamine and serotonin. Serotonin and dopamine are called the feel good neurotransmitters as they control mood. These two neurotransmitters work in concert and need to maintain a balance in the brain. Theanine appears to help preserve this balance.

When researchers began looking into the effects of theanine they wondered about the differences between coffee and green tea consumption. Both beverages contain almost equal amounts of caffeine; while coffee drinkers suffer the stimulating effects of caffeine, green tea consumers do not. It was determined theanine in green tea mediates the effects of caffeine.

L-T produces a tranquilizing effect in the brain without causing drowsiness or dull feelings. In fact research has shown that theanine increases the incidence of alpha waves in the brain. Of the four different types of brain waves, alpha waves denote a relaxed state of mental alertness. This is the mental state meditation brings about.

Twenty to thirty minutes after taking theanine in capsule form, you feel the alpha state begin as muscles relax and the brain changes gears. Theanine stimulates the production of alpha waves, directly signaling the brain to relax and yet still feel mentally alert. Theanine promotes a relaxed state of being while increasing concentration and focus.

For almost immediate relief from stress we recommend opening two L-Theanine capsules and pouring them into four or five ounces of juice and adding a dropper full of Mag Chlor 85. This cocktail has profound effects, inducing a calm, relaxed state in minutes. Although theanine does not cause sleepiness, using this combination 30 minutes before bedtime relaxes the mind and body allowing you to gently drift off to sleep.

Research from the University of Shizuoka in Japan suggests L-Theanine may also have applications in controlling hypertension, enhancing learning ability, increasing mental acuity, and improving concentration as well as supporting the immune system.

Antidepressants, benzodiazepines and pain medications seriously deplete natural brain chemicals. The resulting deficiency causes depression, anxiety, and sleeplessness. Theanine's ability to help balance brain chemistry makes it an important supplement when coming off any psychiatric medication. Theanine is safe to use while you are still on medications to rebuild vital neurotransmitters. For more information about this new and extremely versatile amino acid and green tea, read Dr. Sahley's book, *Theanine, The Relaxation Amino Acid.*

Magnesium

Magnesium is such an important mineral we want to take some time to fully explain its benefits. Magnesium can be classified as life's most important mineral; it is essential in 350 enzyme reactions and indirectly required for thousands of others. Without adequate magnesium our metabolic processes (life processes) suffer. Magnesium and B6, or Pyridoxal 5'Phosphate (P5'P for short), must be present or the body cannot assimilate and properly use amino acids. Despite it's importance, different sources report 80 to 90% of the population is magnesium deficient.

Magnesium is considered the number one stress mineral, and plays an important roll in controlling anxiety. When we are under stress, whether mental or physical, our bodies require even higher levels of magnesium. The release of stress hormones causes a huge rise in magnesium dependent reactions; this quickly uses up magnesium stores. Living under continual stress causes magnesium deficiency, which puts the body under more stress creating a vicious cycle.

Feeling tired, run down? Consider your magnesium levels. All living things, plants and animals require a continual supply of energy in order to function. We obtain our energy from the foods we eat, but before the energy can be used, it must first be transformed into a useable form. Adenosine triphosphate (ATP) is the usable form of energy our body makes. ATP is the molecule responsible for storing and releasing all the body's energy. It could be compared to life's batteries, charging and discharging the energy our body needs to support life. Magnesium is essential in this process. When magnesium levels are low, it is impossible for the body to produce adequate energy.

While calcium is essential for muscle contraction, magnesium is needed for muscle relaxation. The body has 657 muscles that need magnesium every second of every day. The heart, our body's most important muscle, contracts and relaxes thousands of times per day. Without sufficient magnesium the heart can go into spasm costing you your life. Research has shown that when a person has a heart attack, if their magnesium levels are low they are more likely to die than those who have adequate magnesium.

Sherry Rogers, M.D. reported in her May/June 1995, *Total Health & Wellness Letter*, a study conducted to evaluate magnesium levels and the incidence of morbidity in heart attacks. A total of 22 patients who were admitted with cardiac arrest had serum magnesium levels drawn immediately. When the data was analyzed later, they found the patients who entered with low magnesium levels were unable to be resuscitated; 100% of the patients with low serum magnesium died.

If you suffer from allergies, you are familiar with how the body reacts to too much histamine. However, few of us realize magnesium deficiency causes release of excess histamine. People with abnormally high amounts of histamine often demonstrate a history of psychiatric problems ranging from mild to severe. People with chronic pain and fibromyalgia demonstrate high histamine levels represented by joint swelling. High histamine levels are often seen in patients with obsessive-compulsive disorders, depression, and phobias.

Calcium has received much attention for the treatment of osteoporosis but magnesium is just as important for bone strength. After age 35 bone loss begins to occur; once women enter menopause the decline in bone mass is rapid leading to osteoporosis and bone fractures. Research shows fewer fractures occur in women supplementing with both magnesium and calcium than in women supplementing only calcium.

Supplementing with magnesium is safe, and essential. People with kidney problems or impaired kidney function should not supplement with magnesium without consulting with a physician. Magnesium can cause loose stools, or diarrhea, in some people. If this occurs, instead of taking all your magnesium once or twice a day, try taking smaller doses, spreading them out over three or four times

Symptoms of Magnesium Deficiency

- Anxiety
- Panic attacks
- Mitral valve prolapse
- Hypertension
- Chronic pain
- Back and neck pain
- Muscle spasms
- Migraines
- Fibromyalgia
- Spastic symptoms
- Chronic bronchitis, emphysema
- Vertigo (dizziness)
- Confusion
- Depression
- Psychosis
- Noise sensitivity
- Ringing in the ears
- Irritable bowel syndrome
- Cardiovascular disease
- Cardiac arrhythmias
- Atherosclerosis/ Intermittent claudication
- Raynaud's disease (cold hands and feet)
- TIA's (Transient ischemic attacks-strokes)
- Constipation
- Fatigue
- Diabetes
- Hypoglycemia
- Asthma
- Seizures
- Kidney stones
- Premenstrual syndrome
- Menstrual cramps
- Osteoporosis

throughout the day, or try a different form of magnesium. Although magnesium comes in many forms, we have found magnesium chloride is the best-tolerated form. Mag Link is an enteric-coated capsule containing magnesium chloride or Mag Chlor 85 is liquid magnesium chloride.

Eating a diet high in refined carbohydrates and processed foods increases the body's requirement for magnesium. The recommended daily value (RDV) for magnesium is 400 mg. The typical American diet provides between 200-300 mg daily. Dr. Mildred Seelig, a nationally recognized magnesium expert, estimates 80% of the population is magnesium deficient. Ingestion of soft drinks and processed foods—all high in phosphates—cause loss of magnesium via the kidneys. Alcohol usage depletes magnesium, as do certain medications; diuretics and asthma medications such as theophylline are known to cause magnesium loss. Diabetics, people who lose fluid through sweating, and anyone over 40 have increased need for magnesium.

Supplementing with magnesium is essential when coming off prescription medicines, alcohol or illegal drugs; use of these products depletes magnesium levels. Magnesium deficiency interferes with ability to sleep, causes irritability, increased muscle pain, low energy, and depression.

Taurine

The biological significance of taurine is now recognized by a growing number of nutritional and neurological researchers. Strong evidence suggests that this important amino acid is an essential dietary compound for humans and that deprivation of the newborn of a dietary source of taurine may have deleterious results. Taurine is needed for normal development and health of the central nervous system. Disturbances in taurine metabolism are seen in problems as diverse as epilepsy and heart disease.

Taurine is a naturally occurring amino acid that does not occur in proteins. Taurine is found in appreciable concentrations in the brain, and more taurine is found in the brain than in other tissues. Taurine protects and stabilizes the brain's fragile membranes and acts as a neurotransmitter. Only in the last couple of years has taurine been added to the growing list of neurotransmitters. Taurine seems to be closely related in its structure and metabolism to other neurotransmitters such as glycine and GABA. Taurine, like GABA, is inhibitory.

Taurine, or a modified taurine, may someday supersede synthetic tranquilizers. Research is now in progress. Anti-seizure activity in epilepsy has been demonstrated with taurine intakes between 200 and 1,500 milligrams per day, although intakes as high as 7,000 milligrams have been used.

Taurine also plays an important part in bile formation, and thus, is important to fat metabolism and blood cholesterol control. This could prove very helpful in the alcoholic or sugar addict for fat metabolism and liver function.

In many mammals, taurine is synthesized from L-cysteine. However, in man, the bulk of the taurine is derived from dietary sources or produced from cysteine. An outstanding dietary source of taurine is animal/fish protein and marine animals, especially oysters, clams, mussels, and snails.

Taurine is the second most prevalent inhibitory neurotransmitter in the brain. When withdrawing from medications or drugs, taurine helps to reduce muscle pain, tremor, and shaking. It also calms the mind.

Lithium

Lithium research has demonstrated this element has multiple neuroprotective properties in the brain. Lithium provides a large degree of protection against brain damage characteristic of various neurodegenerative diseases. The action of lithium in the brain is antioxidant; it is able to detoxify toxic substances known as free radicals. Lithium's mechanism of action on the brain is still unknown but research does support its effect on the neurotransmitters, serotonin and norepinephrine.

There is growing evidence lithium may be an essential mineral in the human diet. Animals on low lithium diets have shown reproductive problems, shorter life spans, poor lipid metabolism and behavioral abnormalities. Researchers, using data collected over ten years from 27 counties in Texas, found the incidence of homicide, rape, and suicide were significantly higher in counties whose drinking water contained little or no lithium compared to counties with higher lithium.

Lithium orotate, a naturally occurring mineral, is the treatment of choice for recurring bipolar disorder, serving as an effective mood enhancer in 75 to 85% of bipolar patients. Lithium orotate offers both short and long-term benefits for the health of the nervous system. According to Jonathan Wright, M.D., lithium orotate is safe, in fact desirable, to use with other patent medications, as it will protect brain cells against the drugs unwanted toxic effects.

Research reported in the *Journal of Alcohol* (1986) demonstrated lithium orotate was of benefit in the treatment of alcoholics, as well as useful in alleviating alcohol-related symptoms of liver dysfunction, seizure disorders, chronic headaches, hyperthyroidism, seasonal affective disorder and Meniere's syndrome.

Lithium orotate is 20 times more bioactive than other lithium salts, this allows for lower doses reducing the toxic effects of prescription lithium. The recommended dose is one capsule twice daily with meals. This provides 4.8 mg of elemental lithium from each 120 mg capsule. This provides one to two percent of the dose provided by prescription forms of lithium.

Lithium is neither a tranquilizer nor sedative. Lithium does not drug the person or cause them to be sluggish or sleepy. What lithium does is normalize the mood of a manic person—decreasing bouts of mania and moderating periods of depression. The biochemical affects of lithium within the body are wide spread because the gastrointestinal tract immediately absorbs and transports it to every tissue in the body. Lithium stays in the tissues for 24 hours before being excreted by the kidneys.

According to Jonathan Wright, M.D., if you are taking lithium on a regular basis you should also take essential fatty acids (EFAs) and Vitamin E daily. Dr. Wright goes on to say researchers have reported lithium may actually help repair abnormally functioning signaling pathways in critical areas of the brain.

Lithium alters the body concentrations of both sodium and potassium. Lithium controls the excretion rates for both of these basic biological ions as well as the hormones that control the body's electrolyte balance. Lithium is now being considered an anti-aging nutrient for the brain by protecting it against toxic influence.

The future of natural lithium is vast and will continue to present many benefits to those who research it as well as those who take it daily.

Ester C

Vitamin C is important in the treatment of anxiety, stress, depression, and pain. Vitamin C detoxifies drugs from the body and helps to neutralize withdrawal symptoms. Vitamin C is essential in rebuilding the liver, adrenals, and the immune system. Regular Vitamin C, ascorbic acid, is very acidic, and can cause gastrointestinal upset in high doses. G.I. upset can further deplete magnesium and calcium. The best form of C to use is Ester C.

In 1987, clinical studies established that Ester C Polyascorbate is totally neutral, having a pH of 7.0. It does not cause gastrointestinal upset or diarrhea. Studies show that Ester C is four times more bioavailable than ordinary vitamin C.

Ester C is a unique complex mixture with a distinctive molecular personality. This form of vitamin C is more available to the tissues of the body, and is available within 20 minutes after ingestion, and 24 hours later, some of it is still there. Ordinary vitamin C is out of the body within 4 hours after ingestion; even time-release vitamin C has been excreted while the Ester C is still working and available to the body.

All humans, adults, and children need vitamin C, and they need it daily. Ester C has been extremely effective in our detoxification program. At The Pain & Stress Center, we use varying doses for adults in detoxification ranging from 2,000 to 10,000 mg daily.

Melatonin

Melatonin, a neurohormone, is produced in the pineal

gland, a tiny gland at the base of the brain. The pineal gland resembles a pinecone in shape, and is about the size of a pea.

In the evening hours, the pineal gland reacts to diminishing levels of daylight. It starts producing and releasing melatonin into the blood flowing through the body making you drowsy. The secretion of melatonin peaks in the middle of the night during your heaviest hours of sleep. In the morning, bright light shining through the eyelid reaches the pineal gland, which reacts by switching off the production of melatonin removing the sleep state.

The pineal gland is connected to the rest of the hormonal system, and melatonin production influences the functioning of other hormones in the body. During darkness and sleep, melatonin modifies the secretion of hormones from the pituitary gland. The pituitary gland is the master gland of the hormonal system; regulating the secretion of hormones controlling growth, metabolism, thyroid and the adrenal gland.

Since the duration of daylight changes both daily and seasonally, melatonin effectively tells the cells in the body the time of day and year. Melatonin controls the circadian rhythm in the body. The circadian rhythm has a central role in the energy involved in all metabolic processes such as the sleep-wake cycle. Research conducted at M.I.T. and released in February 1994 showed small amounts of melatonin can bring on sleep without the narcotic effect of drugs. For best results melatonin should be taken an hour or two before bed. People under 30 years of age should use Melatonin in very low doses, ranging from 0.5 to 1.0 mg; if over forty use 1.5 to 3 mg an hour before bedtime. Consult a health care professional for exact dosing.

Sleep Link

Insomnia is one of the top complaints from people when discontinuing medications and drugs. Many psychiatric drugs used today disrupt normal sleep patterns and it can take months to reestablish them according to *Psychiatric Annals* (Vol. 25, No. 3, March 1995). Adequate sleep is critical to physical and mental health as anyone who has missed even one night of sleep can attest to. The inability to sleep can be a sizable roadblock to discontinuing medications.

Sleep Link, a unique blend of neuronutrients, can be the answer to rebalancing brain chemicals. Sleep Link supplies the brain with amino acids and herbs that restore natural brain chemicals needed for sleep.

Melatonin combined with 5-HTP balances the circadian rhythm, our internal biological clock that helps the body become sleepy at the appropriate time. GABA cools the brain and shuts down the emotionally loaded limbic system. L-Theanine relaxes the body, reducing muscle tension so you can sleep restfully. Ashwagandha acts as a sedative and induces relaxation. Passion Flower, a sedative-hypnotic herb, prepares the brain and body for sleep. GABA, glutamine, and glycine function as inhibitory neurotransmitters; they help the brain to slow down enabling sleep.

Ashwagandha

Ashwagandha (Withania somnifera) is a shrub grown in India and North America. Its roots have been used for thousands of years by practitioners of Ayurvedic medicine, an ancient medical practice from India. Ashwagandha is traditionally used to *balance life forces,* as anti-stress or an adaptogen; a promoter of good health. In herbal medicine an adaptogen is any substance that helps the body to adapt and protect it from biological, chemical, and physical stressors.

Over 35 active chemicals have been identified in ashwagandha. Ashwagandha's most active principles (alkaloids, withanolides, and withaferins) are similar to those of ginseng, but where ginsing is stimulating, ashwagandha appears to have a calming effect. Withanolides and withaferins in ashwagandha have anti-inflammatory, antioxidant, and antimicrobial actions that contribute to support of the immune system. Somniferine, another chemical found in ashwagandha, has hypnotic (sedative) properties, and promotes deep, dreamless sleep.

Ashwagandha is classified as a *tonic* or adaptogenic herb enhancing the immune system. Ashwagandha has been used to treat anemia, inflammation, stress, bacterial infection, and diarrhea. In India Ashwagandha is used for impotence, sterility, and premature ejaculation. Studies done in India show that ashwagandha increases sperm counts. In women, it treats sterility and increases fertility. At the Pain & Stress Center we have found that Ashwagandha helps reduce symptoms associated with menopause, especially the sleep disturbance. Like ginsing, ashwagandha is considered to be an anti-aging herb.

Along with the positive impact on bodily functions, ashwagandha has important effects in the brain. Researchers from the University of Leipzin in Germany, found ashwagandha increases acetylcholine receptor activity when tested in rats. The researchers say, "The drug-induced increase in acetylcholine receptor capacity might partly explain the cognition-enhancing and memory-improving effects of extracts from Withania somnifera observed in animals and humans." In India ashwagandha is administered for treatment of senile dementia and Alzheimer's disease. A 2002 laboratory study indicates ashwagandha stimulates the growth of axons and dendrites in the brain.

The University of Texas Health Science Center Department of Pharmacology conducted a study in 1991 that indicated extracts of ashwagandha had GABA-like activity. This may account for the herb's anti-anxiety effects.

Animal studies demonstrate that ashwagandha relaxes smooth muscle tissue giving relief from stress and muscle tension.

At the Pain & Stress Center we have found ashwagandha (Mellow Mind) helps patients when coming off prescription medications. Ashwagandha's calming effects on the central nervous system make it perfect to counteract the hypersensitivity seen in medication withdrawal. Ashwagandha is also an effective sleep aid, especially when coming off sleep medications or benzodiazepines.

Essential Fatty Acids

Essential fatty acids refer to fats that must be provided by the diet. Dietary fat has received a great deal of bad press over the years causing us all to scurry around looking for fat-free foods. Many of these foods are highly processed foods that do not create optimum health.

The other end of that spectrum is the *Atkins* type diet where high protein along with high fat content is recommended. All this ends up being very confusing, but the truth is, fat is an essential dietary element. As the major component of the brain, it is vital to our health, both mental and physical.

The key to fat health is the types and correct balance. The brain is composed of 60% fat, and is especially dependent on specific fats. When the correct fats are not present in the proper amounts, the brain substitutes substandard fats for its needs. This leads to problems of poor mental health such as depression, addictions, bipolar disorder, and attention deficit disorder. Supplying the brain with DHA, an omega-3 fatty acid can have profound effects on mood and brain function.

Fats are either saturated or unsaturated and come from plant and animal sources. From a nutritional view, they are called fatty acids. The essential fatty acids (EFAs) linoleic acid (LA) and alpha-linolenic acid (ALA) are the major building blocks of fats. They are considered essential because our bodies cannot synthesize them and they must be provided through the diet. Linoleic acid is commonly found in most plant oils (sunflower, safflower, canola, and corn), and nuts, seeds, and soybeans. Alpha-linolenic acid is found in the oils of flax, hemp, walnut, and green leafy vegetables. Both LA and ALA are polyunsaturated fats.

Fatty acids are categorized by an omega designation; the omega-6 and omega-3 oils are what we are concerned with in brain function. LA and ALA are the precursors, or parent fatty acids for the ones listed below.

Fatty Acids

Omega 6 Fatty Acids	Omega 3 Fatty Acids
Linoleic Acid (LA)	Alpha-Linolenic Acid (ALA)
Gamma-Linolenic Acid (GLA)	Eicosapentaenoic Acid (EPA)
Arachidonic Acid (AA)	Doxosahexaenoic Acid (DHA)

The body needs these two EFAs to be provided in balance. Our ancestors consumed diets high in both omega-6 fats (from seeds and nuts) and omega-3 (plants and game). Scientists estimate their consumption of these fatty acids was in a ratio of 1:1 to a maximum of 4:1. The common diet eaten today is top heavy due to over-consumption of omega-6 fats and trans fatty acids; this is reflected by a ratio as high as 20 or 30:1. Dr. Donald Rudin, author of *The Omega-3 Phenomenon*, estimates we have reduced our omega-3 fatty acid consumption by 80%. This decrease in omega-3 fatty acids directly correlates to the rise in depression, attention deficit disorder (ADD), bipolar disorder, as well as every chronic disease prevalent today.

Linoleic acid and alpha-linoleic acid form the basis of the immune systems pro-inflammatory and anti-inflammatory chemicals; our current dietary imbalance throws us into a state of constant inflammation. Scientists are now saying persistent inflammation is the underlying cause of every chronic disease we face today. The choice of oils we eat impacts our health from heart disease, diabetes, allergies, obesity, arthritis to Alzheimer's disease.

This imbalance of fats greatly impacts our brain health. Remember, 60% of our brain is composed of fats. Of that, nearly one third are polyunsaturated and must be derived from our diet; in other words, they must come from the two-parent oils, linoleic acid and alpha-linolenic acid.

Little linoleic or alpha-linoleic acid is found in the brain. The brain prefers two other fatty acids called arachidonic acid (AA) an omega-6 fatty acid, and docosahexaenoic acid (DHA) an omega-3 fatty acid. DHA can be produced in the body from the essential fatty acid alpha-linolenic acid (ALA). Researchers tell us that at best, only about 15% of consumed ALA can be converted to DHA. For most of us, our high intake of linoleic acid from corn, canola, and other vegetable oils prevents this conversion; so little, if any, ALA actually converts to DHA. This leaves our brains to function on inferior fatty acids. While most authorities believe flax seeds and oils are important for other reasons, they are not a good source of DHA. DHA can be obtained directly from cold-water fish such as salmon, mackerel, herring, sardines, and anchovies or from fish oil supplements. DHA is critical in fetal brain development and infancy. Research has shown children who have adequate levels of DHA have higher IQ's and better visual acuity than children with low levels. Supplementing DHA shows positive results in children with attention deficit disorder (ADD).

DHA plays a critical role in parts of the brain that require a high degree of electrical activity. The synapse is the gap between neurons. The synapse is where one nerve ending communicates with another and is the place where the neurotransmitters work. Other areas of high DHA

The Synapse

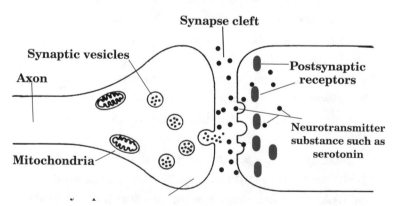

The Synapse separates nerve cells. The synaptic vesicles contain neurotransmitters in reserve until an impulse triggers the release of the neurotransmitters so the message transmits to the next neuron. This process happens in a split second and allows our cells to talk to each other.

concentration are the photoreceptors of the retina, the mitochondria of nerve cells, and the cerebral cortex, the outer layer of the brain. As mentioned earlier, if DHA is not present in adequate amounts, the brain is required to use inferior oils for this vital work.

DHA is essential to proper brain functioning. Deficiencies of total omega-3 fatty acids and lower omega-3 to omega-6 ratio are found in patients with Alzheimer's disease, other dementias, and in cognitive impairment associated with aging. Low serum DHA is a significant risk factor for development of Alzheimer's disease.

DHA levels have a direct effect on mood. Historically cultures where fish is eaten regularly have low levels of depression. There appears to be a direct correlation between depression and the balance of omega-6 to omega-3 ratios. Julia Ross, M.A., author of *The Mood Cure*, says "Omega-3 essential fatty acids are a spectacular good-mood food." Many long-standing depressions have suddenly improved with the addition of this one simple nutrient. Studies show supplementing with DHA raises dopamine, an important neurotransmitter implicated in depression levels by up to 40%.

Based on all the scientific evidence, DHA is an important supplement for everyone regardless of age. DHA and EFAs are vital nutrients for anyone who wants to stop taking antidepressants, pain medications, or is detoxing from alcohol because of their mood enhancing capabilities.

Note of Caution about DHA & Fish Oils: Be very careful with the quality of DHA and fish oils, as some are very high in mercury and other heavy metals. The body does not easily remove heavy metals. Over time, these metals build-up in the body.

11
Withdrawal Support

Nutritional Support For
SSRI Withdrawal

Brain Link – 2 to 3 scoops in morning in juice, *OR* **SBNC** (Super Balanced Neurotransmitter Complex), 2 capsules in the morning and 2 in the evening.

T-L Vite – 1, every evening with main meal. If you take Brain Link, you do not need to take T-L Vite.

B Complex – 1 every morning with breakfast. (Do not take if you are taking Brain Link.)

Decaffeinated Green Tea Extract – 1 (500 mg) capsule with lunch.

DLPA 750 – 1 in morning and 1 in evening. (Do not take if you are taking Brain Link.)

Anxiety Control - 2 capsules, three times per day, divided.

Mag Link 4 to 6 per day, divided. Dosage should be adjusted to individuals bowel tolerance. If loose stools or diarrhea occur, decrease by 1 capsule, or spread further apart.

Mag Chlor 85 – can be used instead of Mag Link. Take 25 drops (one dropper full), two to three times per day.

L-Theanine – 2 capsules, twice daily.

Liquid Serotonin – 10 to 15 drops three times per day. Use between doses of L–T to quickly calm your nerves.

Rodex B6 (150 mg timed-release cap) – 1 in the morning.

HTP10 - 1 to 3 capsules, 30 minutes prior to bedtime *OR* use the *Night Sleep cocktail*. To mix the Night Sleep cocktail, open 2 L–T and dissolve in small amount of water.

Then, add juice and 15 to 20 drops of Mag Chlor 85.

Mobigesic – 1 or 2 tabs, every four to six hours as needed for tension headaches or pain.

72 Hours After You Stop A SSRI

Anxiety Control – 2 in the morning, 2 in the afternoon, 2 in the evening.

Mag Link – Continue 4 to 6 per day, divided.

5-HTP (50 mg) - 1 morning, 1 afternoon, 1 bedtime.

Rodex B6 - 150 mg in morning.

Mobigesic – 1 or 2 tabs, every four to six hours as needed for tension headaches or pain.

Decaffeinated Green Tea Extract – 1 (500 mg) capsule with lunch.

After 2 weeks, change from 5-HTP to Mood Sync. Use 1 or 2 capsules of Mood Sync, three times per day and 5-HTP (50 mg) 1 to 2 capsules at bedtime. This combination helps maintain your serotonin level and gives you a feeling of well-being.

Nutritional Support For Tricyclic (TCA) or MAO Antidepressant Withdrawal

Brain Link – 2 to 3 scoops in morning in juice, *OR* **SBNC** (Super Balanced Neurotransmitter Complex), 2 capsules in the morning and 2 in the evening.

T-L Vite – 1, every evening with main meal. If you take Brain Link, you do not need to take T-L Vite.

B Complex – 1 every morning with breakfast. (Do not take, if you are taking Brain Link.)

Decaffeinated Green Tea Extract – 1 (500 mg) capsule with lunch.

DLPA 750 – 1 in morning and 1 in evening. (Do not take if you are taking Brain Link.)

Anxiety Control - 2 capsules, three times per day, divided.

Mag Link 4 to 6 per day, divided. Dosage should be adjusted to individual's bowel tolerance. If loose stools or diarrhea occur, decrease by 1 capsule, or spread further part *OR* **Mag Chlor 85** – can be used instead of Mag Link. Take 25 drops (one dropper full), two to three times per day.

L-Theanine – 2 capsules, twice daily.

Decaffeinted Green Tea Extract (500 mg) – 1 capsule at noon.

Liquid Serotonin – 10 to 15 drops three times per day. Use between doses of L–T to quickly calm your nerves.

Rodex B6 (150 mg timed-release cap) – 1 in the morning.

Melatonin 3 mg - 1 at bedtime. (Note: If you experience vivid dreams or nightmares, reduce your mg dosage of melatonin. If you prefer, use the *Night Sleep Cocktail* (see on previous page).

Mobigesic – 1 or 2 tabs, every four to six hours as needed for tension headaches or pain.

72 Hours After You Totally Stop The Tricyclics (TCA) Or MAOs

Mood Sync – 1 to 2 caps in morning and afternoon.

B Complex Capsule – 1 capsule in morning.

5-HTP (50 mg) – 1 or 2 capsules, 30 minutes prior to bedtime.

Anxiety Control –2 in the morning and 2 in the afternoon.

Decaffeinated Green Tea Extract (500 mg) – 1 capsule per day with noon meal.

Liquid Serotonin – 10 to 15 drops (1 dropperful) under the tongue as needed for anxiety.

Tyrosine 850* – 1 capsule, twice daily for chronic depression. **Warning: Do not mix tyrosine with MAOs or tricyclic antidepressants, or if you have had cancerous melanoma.*

Mag Link 4 to 6 per day, divided. Dosage should be adjusted to individuals bowel tolerance. If loose stools or diarrhea occur, decrease by 1 tablet or spread further apart.

Rodex B6 (150 mg timed release capsule) – 1 in morning.

Nutritional Support For Hypnotic (Sleep Meds) Withdrawal

Brain Link – 2 to 3 scoops in morning in juice, *OR* **SBNC** (Super Balanced Neurotransmitter Complex), 2 capsules in the morning and 2 in the evening.

T-L Vite – 1, every evening with main meal. If you take Brain Link, you do not need to take T-L Vite.

B Complex – 1 every morning with breakfast. (Do not take, if you are taking Brain Link.)

Decaffeinated Green Tea Extract – 1 (500 mg) capsule with lunch.

*Use **either** the Anxiety Control, Mood Sync OR L–T. You do not need to take all three!*

Anxiety Control – 2 capsules, two to three times per day, divided.

L-Theanine – 2 capsules, twice to three times daily.

Mood Sync* - 1 or 2 capsules, twice daily. *See warning previous page under Tyrosine.*

Mag Link – 4 to 6 per day, divided. Dosage should be adjusted to individual's bowel tolerance. If loose stools or diarrhea occur, decrease by 1 capsule, or spread further apart.

Mag Chlor 85 – can be used instead of Mag Link. Take 25 drops (one dropper full), two to three times per day.

Decaffeinted Green Tea Extract (500 mg) – 1 capsule at noon.

Liquid Serotonin – 15 drops (1 dropper squeeze), three times per day.

Mellow Mind – 1 or 2 capsules at bedtime as needed for sleep. *Do not use Mellow Mind until you have stopped taking the medication.*

Nutritional Support For Pain Drug Withdrawal

Use same withdrawal reduction schedule as for benzodiazepines reducing one-fourth (¼th) of total dosage per week.

Anxiety Control - 2, three times per day.

DLPA 750* – 1 to 2 capsules in the morning, afternoon, and evening. If needed, take 2 more in the middle of the night. *Warning: Do not mix DLPA with MAOs or tricyclic antidepressants, or if you have had cancerous melanoma. Take DLPA with food, if you have hypertension (high blood pressure).*

Mag Link - 2, twice to three times per day, divided. Adjust dosage to your bowel tolerance. If loose stools or diarrhea occur, decrease by 1 capsule, or try spacing further apart. **OR Mag Chlor** – use instead of Mag Link. Take 10 to 25 drops (one dropper full), two to three times per day.

Decaf Green Tea Extract – 1 capsule, two times daily.

Brain Link Complex* – 2 to 3 scoops in morning in juice, *OR* 2 **SBNC** (Super Balanced Neurotransmitter Complex*) capsules, twice in the morning and afternoon.

L–T (L-Theanine Complex) – 2 capsules, twice daily.

Taurine – 1 (1000 mg) capsule, twice daily.

B Complex - 1 in morning.

Sleep Link – 1 or 2 capsules, 30 minutes before bedtime, *OR* you can use 2, **5-HTP** 50 mg capsules, 30 minutes prior to bedtime.

Mellow Mind – 1 or 2 capsule(s) (500 mg Ashwagandha) at bedtime, if needed in addition to Sleep Link.

Exercise such as walking, swimming, golf, or tennis daily.

12
Nutritional Support Products

5-HTP (5-hydroxytryptophan) is precursor to serotonin in the body. 5-HTP is about 10 times stronger than tryptophan, and is only one step biochemically away from serotonin.

Tryptophan → 5-HTP → Serotonin (the Master Controller)

Serotonin is the master controller in the brain and body. The gastrointestinal tract has 80% of the receptor sites in the body while the brain has about 5%. Serotonin produces a relaxed, calm, secure, mellow, uplifted, and tranquil mood. Serotonin helps with insomnia, pain, depression, anger, anxiety, and OCD (Obsessive Compulsive Disorder). *NOTE: Do not use if you are taking Selective Serotonin Reuptake Inhibitors (SSRIs) medications or MAO antidepressants.*

Anxiety Control 24 (AC 24) is a unique amino acid support formula. Anxiety Control combines amino acids (GABA, glycine, and glutamine), herbs (Passion Flower and Primula Officinalis), the mineral (magnesium), and essential cofactor, B6. AC decreases anxiety, stress, tension, or other symptoms due to an overstressed mind and body. Anxiety Control contains the major inhibitory neurotransmitters in the brain. Magnesium and B6 are major cofactors for activation of amino acids in the body. The herbs, Passion Flower and Primula Officinalis, are calming herbs that support your overstressed body and quiets the central nervous system naturally. You can use Anxiety Control all day or at night to feed your brain and body.

B Complex is a complex of the "B" vitamins. The B vitamins are important to our nervous system. B6 serves as an activator of amino acids and many enzyme reactions in the body.

Brain Link Complex is a total amino acid complex in powder form that creates the neurotransmitter links for enhanced brain function. You can use Brain Link daily, and it can be used in conjunction with all other supplements. Brain Link is the most complete neurotransmitter formula available on the market today. Brain Link is perfect for all ages, 1 to 100.

Decaffeinated Green Tea Extract contains 500 mg of decaffeinated green tea with 95% polyphenols. This formula provides the benefits of green tea in capsule form.

DLPA (DL-phenylalanine) contains 50% D-and 50% L-phenylalanine. DLPA helps with depression and pain. The D form actually work with the body by extending the lifespan of your endorphins in the nervous system. Endorphins are the the morphine-like chemicals that the brain produces to regulate pain and the transmission of pain signals. *A runner's high* is simply an endorphin release. Endorphins are inhibitory neurotransmitters in the brain and nervous sytem. DLPA helps fight both depression and pain. The use of drugs reduces our endorphins and neurotransmitters. No wonder stress induced pain sufferers are depressed and are low in 34 of the 36 neurotransmitters made from amino acids. *(NOTE: Do not use DLPA (DL-Phenylalanine) if you take MAOs or tricyclic antidepressants, or if you have a history of melanoma or other cancer.)*

Ester C is the best form of Vitamin C available today.

Ester C has a pH of 7 and is extremely gentle on the GI tract. You do not get diarrhea, gas, or upset stomach when you use Ester C. Studies show Ester C works like a timed-release form of Vitamin C and stays in the body for up to 24 hours. Regular Vitamin C is only in the body for 4 hours.

GABA is a major inhibitory amino acids found in the brain and throughout the body. GABA plays a significant role with anxiety, stress, pain, depression, etc. GABA plays an essential role in neuronal and behavior inhibiton; 40 to 50% of the synapses found in the brain contain GABA. GABA's concentration in the brain is about 200 to 1000 times greater than other neurotransmitters such as acetylcholine and norepinephrine. When your GABA level is low, you feel extremely stressed and out of sorts. The greatest concentration of GABA is in the basal ganglia followed by the hypothalamus, hippocampus, cortex, amygdala, and thalamus.

GABA inhibits the cells from firing so less anxiety-related messages reach the cortex. GABA prevents you from becoming overwhelmed from anxiety, panic, or pain.

NOTE: But too much GABA is not good either. You will experience the same symptoms as if you were having a panic or anxiety attack. Other symptoms include numbness and tingling around the mouth, arms or face, shortness of breath, difficulty breathing. If you accidently get too much, do not panic. The feeling will go away in a few minutes. Drink a large glass of water and eat a few soda crackers or other food. Your body is just telling you that you got too much GABA.

Glutamine is a conditionally essential amino acid and is the third most prevalent in the brain and body. Glutamine is an inhibitory neurotransmitter that acts as a precursor for GABA. Glutamine readily crosses the blood brain barrier into the brain where it provides energy and mental alertness. Glutamine strengthens the immune system and is vitally important for your gastrointestinal tract. Glutamine helps heal the intestines with Leaky Gut Syndrome that results from NSAIDs such as aspirin, Motrin, Celebrex, etc., or food allergies. You could not exist if you did not have adequate glutamine.

L–Theanine (L–T) is a new amino acid that promotes total body relaxation. L-Theanine comes from green tea that dramatically effects the release of neurotransmitters such as dopamine, serotonin, and GABA. Theanine increases GABA in the brain and has no side effects or contraindications. You can take L–T as capsules, or open the capsule and put the L–T in water for faster action. L–T increases alpha waves in the brain and calms nervous or anxious activity.

You can combine L–T with GABA and other amino acids. You can use L–T alone or in a combination formula, Sleep Link at bedtime to help you relax so you can sleep. You can combine L–T or Sleep Link with Mag Chlor 85 for a bedtime cocktail that promotes restful, restorative sleep. Simply, open one or two L–T into a small amount of water, then add ten to twenty-five drops of Mag Chlor 85. Add the mixture into a small amount of fruit juice and drink for your bedtime cocktail about 30 minutes prior to bed. If you are using Sleep Link, *do not open the capsule.*

Mellow Mind is 500 mg of Ashwagandha in capsule form. Ashwagandha (Frankincense) has been used since ancient times to promote health and longevity. Ashwagandha contains over 35 active chemicals and is commonly called Indian ginseng. Ashwagandha's most active chemical principles are alkaloids, withanolides, and withaferins. Withanolide and withaferins in ashwagandha have anti-inflammatory, antioxidant, and antimicrobial actions. These special properties support the immune system, fighting inflammation and infections. Somniferine, a chemical found in Ashwagandha, has hypnotic or sedative properties, and promotes deep, dreamless sleep. Somniferine directly affects the central nervous system. Mellow Mind's ashwagandha *(Withania somnifera)* is valued for its anti-aging properties.

Mood Sync is an amino acid formula that combines Tyrosine, GABA, Taurine, Glutamine, 5-HTP, and B6. Mood Sync provides 5-HTP (5-Hydroxytryptophan) that helps elevate the level of serotonin in the brain and body. Tyrosine is the stress amino acid and the precursor to dopamine and norepinephrine. GABA, glutamine, and taurine are inhibitory neurotransmitters that nourish the brain in times of stress, depression, anger, aggression, mood swings, and PMS. *(NOTE: Do not take use if you are taking Selective Serotonin Reuptake Inhibitors [SSRIs] medications.)*

ProDHA is an omega 3 essential fatty acid (EFA), that provides support for the brain and nervous system. ProDHA contains both DHA (dochexaenoic acid) and EPA (eicosapentaenoic acid). Studies show EFAs improve mood and play a major role with depression. EFAs reduce inflammation and pain, and are replacements for the NSAIDs. Be careful with omega 3 EFA fish oils because some are high in mercury and other heavy metals. ProDHA is a purified EFAs fish oil with stabilizing antioxidants and contains no PCBs or heavy metals.

DLPA is a 50% mixture of D and L-Phenylalanine. DLPA increases norepinephrine, dopamine, and allows endorphins to stay in the body longer. *(NOTE: Do not use DLPA (DL-Phenylalanine) if you take MAOs or tricyclic antidepressants, or if you have a history of melanoma or other cancer. Take with food, if hypertensive.)*

Pain Control 24 is a special complex of amino acids and herbs that have special pain-reducing properties. Pain Control contains DLPA, Boswellia, GABA, and Ashwagandha. Pain Control is excellent for reducing stress-induced pain.

Pain Control helps break the stress-tension-pain cycle, and works with chronic conditions also. *(NOTE: Do not use DLPA (DL-Phenylalanine) if you take MAOs or tricyclic antidepressants, or if you have a history of melanoma or other cancer.)*

Sleep Link is an unique product for occasional sleeplessness. Sleep Link contains specific amino acids and herbs that work synergistically to promote restful sleep our brain and body requires to stay healthy. Sleep problems occur when several brain chemical neurotransmittters become out of balance due to stress, anxiety, depression, medications, or diet deficiencies. Sleep Link contains a complex of L–T, melatonin, 5-HTP, GABA, Ashwagandha, Passion Flower, Glutamine, and P5'P (Pyridoxal 5'Phosphate).

Super Balanced Neurotransmitter Complex (SBNC) capsules is a special complex of inhibitory amino acids. Amino acids create neurotransmitters that allow the brain and body to communicate. Our bodies cannot function without neurotransmitters. Super B.N.C. provides your brain with the needed amino acids to enhance maximum use of the brain. An unbalanced diet, anxiety and stress, certain medications plus other factors, contribute to disturbances in amino acid metabolism. Many people are unaware they have impairments of their biochemistry that cause or complicate their health condition. Amino acids are intimately involved in metabolic regulation, and prove very useful as therapeutic agents that reverse the biochemical impairments related to amino acid metabolism. Amino acid therapy is instrumental in correcting or reducing stress and anxiety, chronic fatigue, food and chemical intolerances, frequent headaches, recurrent infections, mental and emotional disturbances, hyperactivity, learning disabilities, neurological disorders, drug cravings, sleeplessness, and eating disorders.

Liquid Serotonin is a special homeopathic 1X formula that contains serotonin in distilled water. You can use Liquid Serotonin for acute anxiety/stress, or to boost the level of serotonin in the brain and body to produce calm and tranquility. Homeopathic formulas work with the body by stimulating the body to produce more serotonin or other neurotransmitters.

Taurine is the second most prevalent amino acid and an inhibitory neurotransmitter in the brain. Taurine reduces muscle pain, tremor, and shaking, and decreases electrical activity (epilepsy) in the brain. Taurine is found in high concentrations in the heart and eyes.

Tyrosine 850 contains 850 mg of pure, pharmaceutical grade L-Tyrosine in capsule form. Tyrosine is the first breakdown step of phenylalanine and is a precursor for the catecholamines, norepinephrine, epinephrine (adrenalin), dopamine, and dopa. Alan Gelenberg, M.D., Department of Psychiatry, Harvard University, found that tyrosine was more effective than antidepressants.

Vitamin E is a fat soluble vitamin that plays an essential roles in the body. Vitamin E is a potent antioxidant and scavenger of free radicals that plays a role in aging. Other roles include anticoagulant, neuroprotector, anti-thrombotic, immune modulator, cell membrane stabilizer, and antiviral activities. Wilfred Shute, M.D. founder of the Shute Institute and Medical clinic, used Vitamin E in the treatment of over 35,000 patients over 40 years. Dr. Shute sums up his experience with Vitamin E, "There is no condition, normal or abnormal, in which Vitamin E is not directly involved. It is, therefore, essential for the normal function of every cell, every tissue, and every organ in the body."

Amino Acid Cofactors

B6 (Pyridoxine) or P5'P

Our bodies cannot function without enzymes, and every chemical reaction within the body starts with the enzyme triggers. Enzyme reactions start with B6 or P5'P (Pyridoxal 5'Phosphate), and serves as a catalyst so the body can digest amino acids (proteins), carbohydrates, and fats. B6 breaks down into P5'P, the biological form of B6. You should take B6 in a timed-release capsule (Rodex B6 150 mg) that releases over 8 to 9 hours, or take P5'P. If you exceed 300 mg of B6 daily, you can develop irreversible neurotoxicity. Using P5'P instead of B6 protects against neurotoxicity, even in children.

Magnesium

Magnesium is an *essential* cofactor in over 300 enzyme and biochemical reactions in the body, and plays an important role in the metabolism of GABA and other amino acids. Magnesium helps to stabilize your nerves and muscles in the brain and body. Up to 70% of Americans are deficient in magnesium, and do not get enough from their diet. If you are low in magnesium, your nerve cells cannot fire correctly and your muscles contract. Magnesium is known as the *stress* mineral and is necessary for energy production and DNA replications, the basis of life. Magnesium is vitally important for anxiety, depression, stress, etc. because it stabilizes the cell membranes. Magnesium is *essential* to your recovery.

Magnesium deficiency causes the release of more histamine that triggers an allergic reaction to a food, chemical, or environmental pollen. Ingestion of soft drinks, alcohol, certain medications, and processed foods that are high in phosphates cause loss of magnesium. Medications such as asthma meds (theophylline), diuretics (lasix), being over 40 years of age, and diabetes increase the loss of magnesium from the body.

The most bioavailable form of magnesium is magnesium chloride. Supplement with magnesium chloride capsules or 85% magnesium chloride liquid such as Mag Link or Mag Chlor 85. Use Mag Link, 3 to 6 capsules per day, divided throughout the day, or Mag Chlor 85, 15 to 25 drops in juice, twice to three times daily, or the amount recommended in our protocols. If loose stools occur, decrease the dose by 1 capsule, reduce the number of drops, or increase the interval between doses. If you have kidney problems, talk to your physician before taking magnesium.

13
Trends In
Substance Abuse

Alcohol

Research reports more than nine million people have a definite problem with alcohol. The past fifteen years have shown a 30% increase in alcohol consumption.

Tobacco

Tobacco is second to alcohol in its widespread use. Fifty-five million Americans smoke cigarettes daily. It is estimated that more than 300,000 people die prematurely each year from illnesses related to smoking. Currently, about 30% of youths and 25% of adults smoke regularly.

Marijuana

Cannabis is the *most commonly used illegal* drug. The rates are highest among 18 to 25 year olds, but its use is spreading to those younger and older. About 12% of high school seniors are daily users. The marijuana that is accessible today can be up to 5 times more potent than the 1970s marijuana. The most common adverse reaction to marijuana is a state of acute anxiety, sometimes accompanied by paranoid thoughts.

Heroin

Heroin is an addictive drug and its use is a serious problem in America. Recent studies suggest a shift from injecting heroin to snorting or smoking because of increased purity and the misconception that these forms are safer. The risk of AIDS and HIV are probably behind this shift. The Drug Abuse Warning Network lists heroin among the three most frequently mentioned drugs reported in drug-related death cases in 2001. Emergency room episodes between 1988 and 1994 increased 64%. In 1992 the use of heroin rose, and is again becoming popular with youths. The 2002 National Household Survey on Drug Abuse (DHSDA) study reports that since mid-1990s, the incidence of lifetime heroin use for youths and young adults increased. In the past year, 404,000 Americans age 12 and over admitted using heroin and 3.7 million divulged using it at least once in their lifetime.

Methadone and Other Opiates

Methadone has become a drug of abuse through its use as a maintenance treatment for about 80,000 users. Since it is effective for about 24 to 36 hours during maintenance therapy, take-home supplies are given to those patients allowed to visit the clinic only two or three times a week. Recently, doctors have prescribed methadone for pain patients.

In 2000, the FDA approved a new drug, Buprenorphine, for the treatment of opiate addiction. Buprenorphine works by partially binding to the mu receptor in the brain and blocks other opiates from binding there also. The mu receptor in the brain is the receptor site in the brain that initiates euphoria. Clinical studies showed that Buprenorphine reduced opiate use and has a low potential for addiction.

Barbiturates

The source of black market barbiturates and other

hypnotics is usually from prescription drugs, but they are supplemented with illegitimately manufactured products.

Minor Tranquilizers

In 1994, more than eighty million prescriptions for minor tranquilizers were filled; this is a reduction from the peak usage of benzodiazepines in 1975. The top five benzodiazepines prescribed in the U.S. are Xanax, Klonopin, Valium, Ativan, and Restoril. Anxiety appears to be the major reason why benzodiazepines are prescribed. One-fourth of all drug-related emergency room visits are connected with tranquilizer usage.

Amphetamines

Amphetamines and other appetite-suppressant prescription drugs accounted for almost eighteen million prescriptions in 1997. Available reports show they were used for attention deficit disorder, narcolepsy, minimal brain dysfunction, and (in short courses) weight control. The level of abuse is holding steady. Amphetamines remain a potential item of increased abuse.

Cocaine

One of the most addictive drugs of abuse is cocaine. Cocaine is a strong central nervous system (CNS) stimulant that potentiates the effect of dopamine in the brain. Dopamine, a neurotransmitter, is associated with pleasure and movement. Dopamine involves the reward system of the brain causing the *high* the cocaine user feels. About 10% of the people who start using cocaine recreationally progress to heavy usage. Cocaine use continues to increase, but most people who indulge do so sporadically. This pattern may be due to its high cost and relative availability. The abuse of this drug is expected to increase during the next few years. In 1996 about 22 million Americans age 12 years and up had used cocaine at least once in their lifetime, 4 million had indulged in the last year, and 1.7 million had snorted cocaine within the past month.

LSD and Other Hallucinogens

LSD, DMT, and other hallucinogenic drugs have declined in use since the mid 1960's, but they have by no means disappeared from the drug scene. Use of PCP or *angel-dust* is on the rise; the results of its ingestion concerns health care professionals and law enforcement officials. The person under the influence of PCP is more apt to engage in unpredictable, violent behavior than has been encountered with other hallucinogens. The individual may present a variety of neurologic and psychiatric toxic reactions that are not easily diagnosed nor treated.

Inhalants

The sniffing of commercial products containing solvents, freon, or the contents of aerosol sprays is a juvenile practice that does not always terminate when one becomes an adult. The practice is on the increase. Sudden sniffing death and chronic organ damage have been documented with the use of aerosol sprays.

The Dangers of Long-Term Psychiatric Drug Use

Consensus in research matters reveals that certain mental states such as depression and schizophrenia are caused in part, by a deficiency of norepinephrine and an excess of dopamine, respectively. Other theories exist about a deficiency of brain internal opiates called endorphins. Deficiency of opiates occur in compulsive disorders such as alcohol and drug-seeking behavior.

The potential for any drug to cause dependence arises whenever the drug changes mood, behavior or perception and from repeated dosages of a drug. The most commonly abused drugs are the opiates, barbiturates, sedative-hypnotics, alcohol, amphetamines, cocaine and other CNS stimulants, and marijuana. Drug dependency properties differ with the drug involved. But, the commonality in all types of drug dependence is psychic dependence. Psychological dependence is the drive or craving requiring repeated administration of a drug to satisfy the craving for pleasure or relief of pain. The other aspect of drug dependence is physical dependence. Withdrawal symptoms are the physical dependence symptoms, which appear when a drug is interrupted or withdrawn. Tolerance is the third property of drug dependence.

Half-life is the amount of time necessary for the body to metabolize or inactivate half the amount of a drug or substance ingested. Half-life usually determines the amount and frequency a drug is given. Withdrawal symptoms are usually predicted by the half-life or elimination rate of a drug, the length of time and the dosage of the drug. Generally, if the half-life is 10 hours, withdrawal symptoms usually occur within 6 to 8 hours of decreased plasma levels. Peak withdrawal symptoms often occur on the second day and decrease by the fourth or fifth day. If a drug has a longer half-life such as Valium, withdrawal symptoms may not start for a week with the peak symptoms occurring during the second week, and by the third or fourth week the symptoms are markedly reduced. Additional long-term symptoms may last for several months.

These symptoms are usually much less intense than the initial withdrawal symptoms.

As an example, the half-life for Clonazapam is 20-80 hours, depending on how often and the amount of drug ingested. Elimination of the drug takes 3 to 5 half-lives for the all the drug to clear the body. In order to eliminate the drug totally from the body the maximum time required would be 5 X 80 hours or about 16 days.

Today, the most dangerous and insidious addictions are the widespread addiction to pharmaceutical drugs. Well-meaning physicians prescribe pharmaceutical medications to people whose system is already out of balance. Millions of otherwise intelligent, responsible people become addicted to chemicals that over time damage physical and emotional health. Prescription drug abuse is one of the most prevalent, yet *least known addiction in the U.S. today.*

Somehow as a culture, we have developed the belief that if a physician prescribes a medication it is safe, non-addictive, and it will improve our health. We are under the illusion that if it has FDA approval, it has been run through a gamut of tests. Think again. The FDA does not perform ANY drug testing. All the testing is done by the pharmaceutical company and submitted to the FDA for approval. The pharmaceutical company can skew the testing to help get the results it wants. This includes throwing people out of studies, controlling the period of the study (so addictive properties are not detected), etc. Don't be fooled. Before starting any prescription drug look at what the drug does, how it works, what the known side effects are, ask questions, don't just blindly follow.

Recently in the *Journal of the American Medical Association (JAMA)*, Dr. Bruce Pomeranz reported over 100,000 Americans die yearly and over two million patients become gravely ill from adverse reactions to prescribed medications. Drug reactions are the sixth leading cause of death in the United States behind heart disease, cancer, stroke, pulmonary disease, and accidents. The risk of having a drug reaction far exceeds other common risks. The risk of a serious side effect from prescription medication is 26%, or 26 out of 100, whereas the risk of a serious car accident is 2%, or 2 in 100. The chance of a serious reaction to a medication is 12 times more likely than a serious car accident. Dr Pomeranz states 1 in 15 hospital patients in the U.S. experience a serious reaction to over-the-counter or prescription drugs, and approximately 5% die from these reactions.

Physicians think they are helping patients by prescribing antidepressants when a patient complains of being down or depressed. An illusion of safety exists about this newest generation of antidepressants, the SSRIs. Doctors have been quick to prescribe them for a variety of problems. When these drugs initially became available, the side effects listed made them seem much safer than MAO and tricyclic antidepressants. However as more and more people have been taking these drugs for years, new and disturbing side effects have surfaced. The FDA has recently required new labeling for all the SSRIs, warning doctors and patients of an increased risk of violence or suicide when beginning these drugs. About 45% of people taking an SSRI report some sexual dysfunction. Authorities believe this number is actually much higher. One of the more disturbing side effects is the difficulty of withdrawing from these medications. Many people are living out a life sentence on medication that is no longer necessary or advisable, but they simply cannot stop the drug.

Antidepressants are the most common class of drugs to produce serotonin syndrome. Serotonin syndrome involves over stimulation of the brain stem and spinal cord producing symptoms of irrational euphoria, headache, seizures, anxiety, agitation and dizziness. Any antidepressant can produce serotonin syndrome. This includes MAOs, SSRIs, and tricyclic antidepressants. All of these drugs have a potential for addiction and abuse. *Do not stop any of these drugs abruptly; follow the detoxification program outlined.* It takes approximately two weeks to clear all Prozac from your body.

Recently, a study done at the University of Pittsburgh Medical Center by Carolyn Cidis Meltzer, M.D. showed serotonin production substantially declines with age. Using a radioactive marker and PET (Positron Emission Tomography) scanning, they evaluated the number and distribution of serotonin receptors in the brains of healthy people ages 18 to 76. The scans showed there is a 55% decline in serotonin receptors in several areas of the elderly person's brain even after normal aging-related changes were taken into account. This may account why older adults have trouble sleeping and why so many are prescribed antidepressants and sleeping medication.

Prescriptions are money for drug companies. The pharmaceutical industry is the *world's number one profit maker!* They have good reason to keep you on a prescription long-term. You weren't born with pharmacological agents in your brain. You were born with natural neurotransmitters that provide communication between the brain cells and body. Each of us is unique and requires a different amount. Amino acid therapy should be tailored to each person's particular needs.

The following are the most commonly prescribed medications for anxiety, depression, pain, insomnia, etc. The drugs are described so you can understand their most common usage, dosage, side effects, interactions with other medications, withdrawal, half-life, etc.

Abilify (brand) ~ Aripiprazole (generic)

Common Usage: Antipsychotic, used in the treatment of schizophrenia.

Action: The mechanism of action is unknown. However, it has been proposed that the efficacy is mediated through a combination of partial agonist activity at dopamine and serotonin receptors.

Common Dosage: The recommended starting and target dose is 10 or 15 mg/day administered on a once-a-day schedule without regard to meals.

Major Side Effects: Flu syndrome, peripheral edema, chest pain, neck pain, neck rigidity, tremor, hypertension, tachycardia, hypotension, bradycardia (pulse < 60), anorexia, nausea and vomiting, ecchymosis (an accumulation of blood under the skin or a bruise), anemia, weight loss, muscle cramps, depression, nervousness, increased salivation, hostility, suicidal thought, manic reaction, abnormal gait, confusion, cogwheel rigidity, dyspnea (difficult, labored, uncomfortable breathing), pneumonia, dry skin, pruritis (itching), sweating, skin ulcer, conjunctivitus, ear pain, urinary incontinence.

Precautions: Abilify has been know to cause *neuroleptic malignant syndrome (NMS)*, a potentially fatal symptom complex], *tardive dyskinesia* (a syndrome of potentially irreversible, involuntary, movements), and *hyperglycemia and diabetes mellitus (in some cases extreme) associated with ketoacidosis, hyperosmolar coma, or death per FDA.*

Interactions with Other Medications: Abilify should not be taken with fluoxetine (Prozac), paroxetine (Paxil), quinidine (antiarrhythmic), carbamazepine (Tegretol), or any medications known to suppress the central nervous system.

Withdrawal: Do not stop this drug suddenly. Check with your pharmacist.

Drug Half-Life: 75 hours for efficient metabolizers (EM) and 146 hours for poor metabolizers (PM).

Adderall (brand) ~ Dextroamphetamine and Amphetamine (generic)

Common Usage: Amphetamine/psychostimulant—Attention Deficit Disorder and Narcolepsy.

Action: Non-catecholamine sympathomimetic amines with CNS stimulant activity.

Common Dosage: A.D.D., 2.5–40 mg per day, divided in two doses. For narcolepsy, 5–10 mg per day, increasing until satisfactory results are obtained.

Major Side Effects: Nervousness, palpitations, agitation, over stimulation, sleeplessness, elevated heart rate and blood pressure, headache, dizziness, dry mouth, insomnia, euphoria, tremor, diarrhea, altered taste sensations, decrease in sexual functioning, loss of appetite, weight loss, itchy skin. Patients with Tourette's syndrome, epilepsy, or any other CNS motor disorders may worsen with Adderall.

Interactions with Other Medications: Avoid alcohol. Ascorbic acid (Vitamin C), fruit juices, or other foods high in acid content decrease absorption of amphetamines. Drugs such as lithium, methenamine (Hiprex), antipsychotics such haloperidol (Haldol) and chlorpromazine (Thorazine), may reduce the effectiveness of Adderall. Drugs high in alkaline content (baking soda, antacids) increase absorption of Adderall. Diuretics such as acetazolamide (Diamox) and hydrochlorothiazide (Hydrodiuril) and other diuretics may augment Adderall and its side effects. Adderall may enhance tricyclic antidepressants such as amitriptyline(Elavil) and imipramine (Tofranil).

166/ Break Your Prescribed Addiction

Amphetamines potentiate analgesic effects of Meperidine (Demerol) and propoxyphene (Darvon, Darvocet). Care must be taken with certain drugs such as Darvon, Fura-zolidone (Furoxone), anti-Parkinson drugs as pergolide (Permax) and carbidopa/levodopa (Sinemet), and some antidepressants as life-threatening situations may result with amphetamine addition. MAO antidepressants such as Nardil and Parnate may potentiate amphetamines in-creasing the release or norepinephrine causing headaches and hypertensive crisis. The effectiveness of medications used for hypertension, heart disease, epilepsy, and glau-coma may be antagonized with the Adderall. OTC drugs containing ephedrine, pseudoephedrine, phenylpropanol-amine, or epinephrine (Sudafed, Dimetapp, Dexetrim) should not be combined with Adderall. Amphetamine-type drugs such as phentermine (Fastin, Ionamin) can cause in-creased blood pressure, heart rate, and other side effects.

Withdrawal: Abrupt withdrawal following high dosages produces extreme fatigue and mental depression. Chronic use and abrupt withdrawal results in severe dermatoses (skin disease without inflammation), marked insomnia, irritability, hyperactivity, and personality changes.

Drug Half-Life: 7–11 hours.

Ambien (brand) ~ Zolpidem (generic)

Common Usage: Hypnotic, short term (7-10 days) in-somnia.

Action: Modulation of GABA.

Common Dosage: 5–10 mg.

Major Side Effects: Drowsiness, dizziness, lightheaded-ness, difficulty concentrating, headache, nausea/vomiting, hangover next morning, muscle and joint pains, upper respiratory infection, lethargy, drugged feeling, and amnesia. Some people have changes in thinking and behavior after using zolpidem. Changes include more aggressive behavior, confusion, loss of personal identity, strange behavior, agitation, hallucinations, worsening of depression, suicidal thoughts.

Interactions with Other Medications: Interaction with alcohol or other CNS depressants may increase side effects.

Withdrawal: Abrupt discontinuation may produce mild depression and restlessness, insomnia, abdominal and muscle cramps, nausea/vomiting, sweating, tremors, convulsions, shakiness, fatigue, flushing, lightheadedness, uncontrolled crying, panic attack, and nervousness.

Drug Half-Life: 1.4–4.5 hours.

Amerge (brand)~ Naratriptan (generic)

Common Usage: Relief for migraine headaches.

Action: Unknown, but believed to bind to $5\text{-HT}_{1D/1B}$ receptors.

Common Dosage: Initially 2.5 mg. If headache returns or partial return, follow with 1-2.5 mg in four hours. Do not exceed 5 mg in 24 hour period.

Major Side Effects: Dizziness, parasthesias, drowsiness, malaise, fatigue, throat/neck symptoms, chest discomfort (including pain, pressure, heaviness, and tightness), feeling strange and burning/stinging sensation, palpitations, abnormal EKGs, ear, nose, and throat infections, thirst, dehydration, fluid retention, sinusitis, upper respiratory inflammation, ringing in ears, vomiting, gastrointestinal pains, muscle pains, stiffness, cramps, sleep disorders, chills/fever, anxiety, depression, sweating, skin rashes and bladder inflammation have been reported after administration. Increased blood pressure, hypersensitivity, coronary artery spasm, cerebral hemorrhage (stroke) have been reported after administration. Serious cardiac events, including some deaths have been reported with Amerge.   These are rare, but may be seen in patients with risk factors predicative of coronary artery disease.

Interactions with Other Medications: If combined with ergot preparations may cause prolonged vasospastic reactions. When combined with SSRIs, weakness, hyper-reflexia, and incoordination may be seen.

Withdrawal: Unknown with short-term use.

Drug Half-Life: 6 hours.

Anafranil (brand) ~ Clomipramine (generic)

Common Usage: Tricyclic antidepressant, treatment of depression, and obsessive-compulsive disorders.

Action: Inhibits reuptake of serotonin in brain and its active metabolite (by-products of the drug as it breaks down) DMCL (desmethylclomipramine) blocks reuptake of norepinephrine in the brain.

Common Dosage: 25-150 mg daily, divided.

Major Side Effects: Drowsiness, dizziness, fatigue, tremors, lowered seizure threshold, blurred vision, fall in blood pressure with standing, dry mouth, constipation, weight gain, excessive sweating, confusion, memory lapses, extrapyramidal symptoms, agitation, skin rash, sun sensitivity, black tongue, nasal congestion.

Interactions with Other Medications: Avoid alcohol and other CNS depressants (alcohol, barbiturates, and benzodiazepines) potent CNS depression.   MAOs may cause hypertensive crisis, hyperpyretic (fever) crisis, severe seizures, rapid pulse > 100, and death.   If amphetamines are added, increase hypertensive and cardiac effects may be seen. Increased blood levels of clomipramine may be seen with the adding of methylphenidate (Ritalin), phenothiazines (Thorazine), haloperidol (Haldol), and cimetidine. Smoking causes increased metabolism of clomipramine. Increased clotting time results when clomipramine is added to warfarin (Coumadin). Adding Levodopa (Sinemet) or phenylbutazone to clomipramine delays absorption of both drugs. Antihypertensive medications are not as effective with the addition of clomipramine. Thyroid medications may increase risk of arrhythmias.

Withdrawal: Abrupt withdraw symptoms following long-term administration include nausea, severe dizziness, malaise, insomnia, and nightmares.

Drug Half-Life: 12–84 hours.

Antabuse (brand) ~ Disulfiram (generic)

Common Usage: Chronic alcoholism.

Action: Antabuse blocks breakdown of alcohol. If the patient ingests even a small amount of alcohol, a very unpleasant reaction (Antabuse-alcohol reaction) occurs.

Common Dosage: 125-500 mg per day.

Major Side Effects: Drowsiness, fatigue, headache, restlessness, nerve pain, blurred or impaired vision, metallic or garlic after-taste, dizziness, insomnia, seizures, delirium, and skin rashes, dermatitis, liver toxicity, blood abnormalities.

Interactions With Other Medications: Alcohol: The Antabuse-alcohol reaction causes flushing, throbbing in head and neck, nausea, copious vomiting, difficulty breathing, sweating, thirst, rapid heartbeats, chest pain, heart palpitations, decreased to low blood pressure, weakness, dizziness, blurred vision, and confusion. Ingestion of a large amount of alcohol can produce severe reactions producing depression, respiratory, cardiovascular collapse, arrhythmias, heart attack, acute congestive heart failure, convulsions, and death. Duration of the reaction varies from 30 minutes to several hours, and varies from person to person usually proportional to amount of Antabuse and alcohol ingested. *Reactions to alcohol may occur up to 14 days after ingesting Antabuse.* Most patients, with even the smallest amount of alcohol, will experience flushing, throbbing, headaches, troubled or rapid breathing, nausea, vomiting, sweating, heart palpitations, fainting, severe weakness, extreme blurred vision and confusion. Larger amounts of alcohol can lead to more serious problems, including seizures, heart attack and death. *It is imperative* that this drug not be given to anyone who has had alcohol of any form 12 hours prior to taking Antabuse including vinegars, cough syrups, mouthwashes, or any liquid medications, prescription or over-the-counter meds containing alcohol. Additionally, any cosmetics (i.e., colognes, after-shaves, lotions or sprays) in which alcohol may be absorbed through the skin, and foods containing alcohol-based sauces or marinades should be avoided. Reactions have been known to occur for as long as up to 12 weeks after the last dose of disulfiram. Disulfiram may make some benzodiazepines such as Valium and Librium increase drowsiness in some patients. Patients on tricyclic antidepressants (such as Elavil, Tofranil, etc.) or metronidazole (Flagyl) may have behavior changes or become confused. Other drugs that might interact with disulfiram are Isoniazid, phenytoin (Dilantin), ethotoin (Peganone), mephenytoin (Mesantoin), and warfarin (Coumadin). Caffeine may enhance certain side effects such as headache, heart palpitations and flushing. Patients allergic to pesticides and rubber (latex) products containing thiuram may have an allergic reaction to this drug.

Aricept (brand) ~ Donepezil (generic)

Common Usage: Treatment of mild to moderate dementia of the Alzheimer's type.

Action: Reversible inhibitor of the enzyme acetylcholinesterase. No evidence exists that donepezil alters the course of the underlying dementing process.

Common Dosage: 5–10 mg daily.

Major Side Effects: Nausea, diarrhea, insomnia, vomiting, muscle cramp, fatigue, hypertension, fecal incontinence, bloating, dehydration, delusions, tremor, irritability, vertigo, aggression, abnormal crying, eye irritation, urinary incontinence and anorexia.

Precautions: Likely to exaggerate muscle relaxation during anesthesia, may cause bradycardia. Monitor patients for gastrointestinal bleeding.

Drug Interactions: None reported.

Drug Half-Life: 70 hours.

Asendin (brand) ~ Amoxapine (generic)

Common Usage: Tricyclic antidepressant—treatment of major depression.

Action: Blocks the reuptake of norepinephrine or serotonin or both in the CNS increasing the concentration of these neurotransmitters as they accumulate in the brain synapses.

Common Dosage: 50-200 mg daily.

Major Side Effects: Drowsiness, dizziness, drop in blood pressure after standing from sitting position, pulse > 100, dry mouth, constipation, urinary retention, weakness, fatigue, confusion, lethargy, memory defects, trouble concentrating, tremors, ringing in ears, extrapyramidal symptoms, skin rash, nausea/vomiting, loss of appetite, diarrhea, abdominal cramps, paralytic ileus, abnormal blood tests, hepatitis, weight gain.

Interactions with Other Medications: Adding MAO inhibitors may create hypertensive crisis, hyperpyretic

crisis (fever > 106°), rapid heartbeats > 100, severe sei-zures, and death. Decreased effects of clonidine and gua-nethidine are seen after the addition of amoxapine.
Avoid alcohol and other CNS depressants (alcohol, bar-biturates, and benzodiazepines) potent CNS depression. If amphetamines are added, increase hypertensive and cardiac effects may be seen. Increased blood levels of amoxapine may be seen when methylphenidate (Ritalin), phenothiazines (Thorazine), haloperidol (Haldol), and cimetidine are added. Smoking causes increased metabo-lism of amoxapine. Increased clotting time results when amoxapine is added to warfarin (Coumadin). Adding Le-vodopa (Sinemet) or phenylbutazone to amoxapine delays absorption of these drugs. Antihypertensive medications are not as effective with the addition of amoxapine. Thy-roid medications may increase risk of arrhythmias.

Withdrawal: Abrupt withdrawal may produce nausea, head-ache, malaise, severe dizziness, insomnia, and nightmares.

Drug Half-Life: 10–50 hours.

Ativan (brand) ~ Lorazepam (generic)

Common Usage: Antianxiety, sedation, benzodiazepine.

Action: Depresses the CNS in limbic system and pro-motes GABA transmission.

Common Dosage: 0.25-6 mg daily, divided.

Major Side Effects: Abuse potential, dizziness, drowsi-ness, CNS depression, memory impairment, headache, weakness, unsteadiness, disorientation, agitation, poor coordination, nausea, change of appetite, sleep distur-bance, blurred vision, dry mouth, skin rash and itching, transient amnesia or memory loss (forgetting events that happen several hours after taking medication), and abnor-mal blood tests.

Interactions with Other Medications: Alcohol and other CNS depressants increase the effects of drugs. Cimetidine increases the sedation of lorazapam.

Withdrawal: Abrupt withdrawal after an extended period of time may produce convulsions, tremor, abdominal and muscle cramps, vomiting, sweating, insomnia, depression, restlessness, anxiety, unhappiness, general dissatisfaction.

Drug Half-Life: 18 hours.

Buspar (brand) ~ Buspirone (generic)

Common Usage: Antianxiety—short-term treatment of anxiety disorders.

Action: Exact mechanism is unknown, but attaches to serotonin and dopamine receptors in CNS.

Common Dosage: 15-30 mg

Major Side Effects: Drowsiness, dizziness, nervousness, insomnia, fatigue, headache, insomnia, dry mouth, weakness, light-headedness, confusion, depression, hypotension (low blood pressure), nausea, skin rash and itching, weight gain/loss, urinary hesitancy/frequency, ringing in the ears, sore throat, nasal congestion, muscle aches, shortness of breath.

Interactions with Other Medications: Adding alcohol, other CNS depressants, sedative-hypnotics, narcotics increase effects of these drugs. In combination with MAO inhibitors, buspirone may elevate blood pressure.

Withdrawal: Abrupt withdrawal may produce gastrointestinal upsets, palpitations, insomnia, and nervousness. Gradual withdraw over at least 2 to 4 weeks is preferred method of withdrawal.

Drug Half-Life: 2–11 hours.

Calan, Isoptin (brand) ~ Verapamil (generic)

Common Usage: Calcium channel blocking agent; antihypertensive, antiarrhythmic, antiangina; used in the treatment of angina, migraine headaches, and bipolar disorders.

Action: Slows the conduction of impulses from atria to ventricles resulting in prolonged refractory (resting period) in heart. This inhibits muscle contraction, vasoconstriction, and cardiac conduction. Mechanism of action in bipolar disorder is unknown.

Common Dosage: 240–480 mg per day in three to four dosages for atrial (cardiac) arrhythmias; 80 mg, three or four daily in bipolar disorders and migraine headaches.

Major Side Effects: Dizziness, headache, fatigue, hypotension (low blood pressure), peripheral edema (swelling in extremities), congestive heart failure, pulmonary edema (fluid in lungs), pulse < 60, constipation, nausea, heart blocks, arrhythmias, rash, dry mouth, diarrhea, urinary frequency, impotence.

Interactions with Other Medications: Increased hypotensive effects with further depression of heart conduction with propranolol (Inderal). Effects of carbamazepine (Tegretol) and theophyllines are increased when verapamil is added. Increased risk of digoxin or digitalis toxicity due to increased plasma levels. Decreased effects of verapamil are seen with Vitamin D, calcium salts, lithium, and rifampin. Interaction of verapamil with nondepolarizing muscle relaxants may increase neuromuscular block. Addition of prazosin, quinidine, and methyldopa yield acute hypotension. Warfarin (Coumadin), sulfonamides, hydantoins, oral hypoglycemics (diabetic meds), and aspirin may produce either increased or decreased plasma levels of these drugs or verapamil.

Withdrawal: Abrupt discontinuation in angina patient may precipitate an increase in length and duration of chest pains.

Drug Half-Life: 4.5-12 hours with repeat dosing.

Catapres (brand) ~ Clonidine (generic)

Common Usage: Antihypertensive—treatment of high blood pressure, ADHD—Attention Deficit Hyperactivity Disorder, tic disorders such as Tourette's syndrome, impulsivity or aggression.

Action: Stimulates receptors in brain stem which results in reduced outflow from CNS and a decrease in vascular resistance in extremities and to kidney, heart rate, and blood pressure.

Common Dosage: 0.2–0.6 mg per day, divided.

Major Side Effects: Sedation, drowsiness, weakness, palpitations, rapid or slow heartbeat, congestive heart failure, nervousness, agitation, nightmares, restlessness, anxiety, hallucinations, delirium, rash, nausea and vomiting, loss of appetite, constipation, malaise, decreased sexual activity, weight gain, muscle or joint pains, dry mouth, dryness of eyes.

Interactions with Other Medications: Clonidine enhances the effects of alcohol, barbiturates, other sedating drugs, digitalis (Digoxin) or calcium channel blockers (Cardizem). If clonidine is combined with a tricyclic antidepressant such as imipramine (Tofranil) or amitryiptyline (Elavil), your blood pressure may increase.

Withdrawal: Abrupt discontinuation of clonidine may cause high blood pressure, headaches, nervousness, tremor, agitation, followed by a rapid rise in blood pressure and elevated catecholamines (adrenaline, norepinephrine). Clonidine should be slowly withdrawn over several days to weeks.

Drug Duration: 8 hours.

Celexa (brand) ~ Citalopram (generic)

Common Usage: Antidepressant

Action: Selective Serotonin Reuptake Inhibitor with minimal effects on the neuronal reuptake of norepinephrine and dopamine.

Common Dosage: 20–60 mg, once daily.

Major Side Effects: Nausea, dry mouth, somnolence, and increased sweating are the most common listed side effects occurring in more than 10% of patients taking Celexa. Other side effects occurring in less than 10% of patients are influenza-like symptoms, nonpathological trauma, pain, postural hypotension, tachycardia, migraine, paresthesia, flatulence, weight decrease, weight increase, abnormal dreaming, aggravated depression, amnesia, apathy, confusion, depression, impaired concentration, increased appetite, sleep disorder, suicide attempt, pruritus, rash, polyuria (frequent urination), and sexual side effects.

Contraindications: Do not use with MAO inhibitors, or within 14 days of discontinuing an MAO.

Cautions: Potential for suicide, and activation of mania. Citalopram has not been tested in patients with seizure disorders. The safety of citalopram during pregnancy and lactation, or patients < 18 years old. has not been established.

Pregnancy: Neonates exposed to Celexa and other SSRIs or SNRI's, late in the third trimester, have developed complications requiring prolonged hospitalization, respiratory support, and tube feeding.

Withdrawal: During research studies abrupt discontinuance of citalopram after eight weeks of use caused incidences of anxiety, emotional indifference, impaired concentration, headache, migraine, paresthesia, and tremor. It is unknown whether gradual discontinuation will prevent these symptoms. It is recommended that the dosage

of citalopram should be tapered off over 1 to 2 weeks.
Drug Half-life: 37 hours.

Clozaril (brand) ~ Clozapine (generic)

Common Usage: Atypical antipsychotic used in the management of severely ill schizophrenic patients.

Action: Binds to dopamine receptors and acts as an antagonist at adrenergic, cholinergic, histaminergic, and serotonergic receptors.

Common Dosage: Begin with ½ of a 25 mg tablet, once or twice daily. Continue with daily dose increments of 25 to 50 mg per day by the end of 2 weeks.

Major Side Effects: Agranulocytosis; seizures; myocarditis; orthostatic hypotension; tachycardia; hyperglycemia and diabetes mellitus; sometimes severe and resulting in coma and death; neuroleptic malignant syndrome; tardive dyskinesia; fever; pulmonary embolism.

Drug Interactions: Should not be used with other drugs having a potential to cause agranulocytosis or otherwise suppress the bone marrow. Should not be taken with benzodiazepines, or any drugs affects the CNS,

Precautions: Increased risk of hyperglycemia and/or diabetes with ketoacidosis, coma, and death associated with use of clozapine.

Withdrawal: Gradual reduction in over a 1 to 2 week period. Closely observe the patient for reoccurrance of psychotic symptoms.

Drug Half-Life: 4–66 hours.

Concerta (brand) ~ Methylphenidate (Extended Release generic)

Common Usage: CNS stimulant; attention deficit hyperactivity disorder; class II controlled drug.

Action: Exact mechanism unknown, but thought to block reuptake of norepinephrine and dopamine.

Common Dosage: 18–54 mg a day, depending on age, weight, and if taking Methylphenidate not in sustained release form. No studies exist on Concerta and children less than 6 years of age.

Major Side Effects: Allergic reaction with difficulty breathing, closing of the throat, or swelling of the lips, unusual behavior or confusion, liver damage, yellowing of the skin or eyes, unusual bleeding or bruising, headache, abdominal pain, dizziness, blurred vision, visual disturbances, tics, anorexia, insomnia, cough, sinusitis, dizziness, nervousness, dyskinesias, hypertension, tachycardia, arrhythmias, Tourette's syndrome, toxic psychosis, seizures, rash, decreased appetite or weight loss or slower weight gain and/or growth.

Interactions with Other Medications: Hypertensive crisis with MAOIs in the last 14 days, tricyclics, SSRIs, dilantin, and coumadin. Use with caution with pressor agents and clonidine. May increase levels of anticonvulsants, coumadin anticoagulants, SSRIs, and tricyclics.

Precautions: Discontinue, if seizures occur. Reduce dose or discontinue, if paradoxical worsening of symptoms occurs. Reassess periodically. Do not use if you have glaucoma, significant anxiety, tension, agitation, or tics or family history or Tourette's. Do not use with GI narrowing, hypertension, heart failure, recent MI (heart attack), hyperthyroidism, psychosis, seizure disorders, depression, normal fatigue states, emotionally unstable. May exacerbate behavior disturbances, thought disorders. Monitor growth, blood pressure, CBC, differential, platelet counts.

Withdrawal: Discontinuing suddenly may produce extreme fatigue, lethargy, increased dreaming, mental depression, and suicidal ideations.

Drug Half-Life: 3.5 hours.

Cylert (brand) ~ Pemoline (generic)

Common Usage: Central nervous stimulant—Attention deficit disorder, narcolepsy.

Action: Central nervous system.

Common Dosage: 37.5 to 75 mg per day.

Major Side Effects: Elevated liver function tests, jaundice, hepatitis, insomnia, nervousness, dizziness, headache, weight loss, nausea, diarrhea, stomach upset, involuntary facial, tongue, or eye movement. Patients with Tourette's syndrome or epilepsy may have increased frequency of tics or seizures. With long-term usage retardation of growth is possible in children.

Interactions with Other Medications: Avoid mixing with alcohol. Do not mix with amphetamines, dexedrine, or didrex. Aggravation of symptoms may be seen with patients taking medications for glaucoma, heart, blood pressure or an enlarged prostate, if pemoline is added. The addition of medications containing ephedrine, pseudoephedrine (cold/allergy remedies), phenylephrine (nose sprays).

Withdrawal: Gradually reduce and taper off dosage over a week.

Drug Half Life: 12 hours.

Darvocet (brand) ~ Propoxyphene and acetaminophen (generic)

Common Usage: Anagesic; relief of mild to moderate pain.

Action: Centrally acting mild narcotic analgesic structurally related to methadone.

Common Dosage: 1 caplet every 4 hours as needed for pain to a maximum of 6. Each tablet contains 100 mg propoxyphene and 650 mg acetaminophen.

Major Side Effects: Dizziness, sedation, nausea and vomiting, constipation, abdominal pain, skin rashes, lightheadedness, headache, weakness, euphoria, dysphoria, hallucinations, and minor visual disturbances.

Drug Interactions: Do not use with other CNS depressants or alcohol.

Precautions: Use with caution to patients with hepatic or renal impairment.

Warnings: Potential for addiction and dependence. Do not prescribe to patients who are suicidal or addiction-prone. Prescribe with caution for patients taking tranquilizers or antidepressant drugs, and patient who use alcohol in excess. Darvocet in excessive doses, either alone ,or in combination with other CNS depressants or alcohol, are a major cause of drug-related deaths; fatalities within the first hour of over dosage are not uncommon.

Withdrawal: If dependant, do not stop suddenly. Reduce slowly.

Drug Half-Life: 6–12 hours.

Depokote (brand) ~ Valproic Acid (generic)

Common Use: Anticonvulsant, prevention of migraine headaches.

Action: Not established, but potentiates GABA in brain.

Common Dosage: 33–110 mg/pound of body weight. If total daily dosage exceeds 250 mg, the dosages must be divided.

Major Side Effects: Nausea, vomiting, drowsiness, dizziness, headache, nausea/vomiting, indigestion, uncoordinated voluntary movement, tremor, weakness, fatigue, personality changes, anxiety, mental depression, skin rash, irregular menses, increased appetite, weight gain, irritability, loss of appetite, diarrhea, constipation, abnormal blood tests, liver failure.

Interactions with Other Medications: Alcohol and other CNS depressants (benzodiazepines) are enhanced with valproic acid. Altered blood levels may be seen with carbamazepine (Tegretol), and phenytoin (Dilantin) causing increased blood serum levels. Aspirin and warfarin

(Coumadin) with valproic acid may increase bleeding times.
Withdrawal: Do not discontinue abruptly. Taper off slowly.
Drug Half-Life: 6–16 hours.

Desyrel (brand) ~ Trazodone (generic)

Common Usage: Antidepressant, treatment of depression and hypnotic for insomnia.
Action: Inhibits serotonin reuptake increasing its concentration at the brain synapse and potentiating its effects.
Common Dosage: 200–600 mg per day, divided.
Major Side Effects: Sedation, drowsiness, dizziness, fatigue, confusion, weakness, tremors, dry mouth, nausea, vomiting, anorexia, hypotension (blood pressure drop when changing from sitting to standing position), sweating, rapid pulse, blurred vision, ringing in ears, urinary retention, skin itching, rash, abnormal prolonged, painful erections in male.
Interactions with Other Medications: The combination of trazodone with alcohol, barbiturates, and other central nervous system depressants increases impairment. Increased levels of digoxin and phenytoin (Dilantin) have been reported with trazodone. Increased bleeding times and bruising may be seen if trazodone is added to Coumadin. It may interact with MAOs.
Withdrawal: After long-term use, abrupt withdrawal symptoms may include headache, nausea, vomiting, muscle pain, and weakness. Trazodone should be discontinued gradually over at least a 2-week period. Depression may return after discontinuation of any antidepressant.
Drug Half-Life: 3–9 hours, average 5 hours.

Dexedrine (brand) ~ Dextroamphetamine (generic)

Common Usage: CNS stimulant—amphetamine; attention deficit disorder and narcolepsy.

Action: Exact mechanism unknown but believed to promote release of norepinephrine in the brain.

Common Dosage: 10–60 mg per day for A.D.D.; 20–30 mg daily in adult narcolepsy.

Major Side Effects: Excitement, overstimulation, restlessness, dizziness, insomnia, euphoria, palpitations, rapid pulse > 100, dry mouth, loss of appetite, weight loss, tremors, headache, symptoms of Tourette's hallucinations, nervousness, blurred vision, elevated blood pressure, cardiac arrhythmias, itchy skin, physical and psychological dependence, inhibits growth in children.

Interactions with Other Medications: Avoid alcohol. Ascorbic acid (Vitamin C), fruit juices, or other foods high in acid content decrease absorption of amphetamines. Drugs such as lithium, methenamine (Hiprex), antipsychotics such haloperidol (Haldol) and chlorpromazine (Thorazine), may reduce the effectiveness of amphetamines. Drugs high in alkaline content (baking soda, antacids) increase absorption of dextroamphetamine. Diuretics such as acetazolamide (Diamox) and hydrochlorothiazide (Hydrodiuril) and other diuretics may enhance dextroamphetamine and its side effects. Dextroamphetamine or other amphetamines may potentiate tricyclic antidepressants such as amitriptyline(Elavil) and imipramine (Tofranil). Amphetamines potentiate analgesic effects of Meperidine (Demerol) and propoxyphene (Darvon, Darvocet). Care must be taken with certain drugs such as Darvon, Furazolidone (Furoxone), anti-Parkinson drugs as pergolide (Permax) and carbidopa/levodopa (Sinemet), and some antidepressants as life-threatening situations may result with amphetamine addition. MAO antidepressants such as Nardil and Parnate may potentiate amphetamines increasing the release or norepinephrine causing headaches and hypertensive crisis. The effectiveness of medications used for hypertension, heart disease, epilepsy, and glaucoma may be antagonized with the amphetamines such as dextroamphetamine. OTC drugs containing ephedrine, pseudoephedrine, phenylpropanolamine, or epinephrine (Sudafed, Dimetapp, Dexetrim) should not be combined with dextroamphetamine. Amphetamine-type drugs such as phentermine (Fastin, Ionamin) can cause increased blood pressure, heart rate, and other side effects. Caffeine in foods and drinks (coffee or colas) increases effects of amphetamines such as dextroamphetamine.

Withdrawal: Abrupt withdrawal following high dosages produces extreme fatigue, mental depression, increased dreaming, lethargy, ideas of suicide. Chronic use and abrupt withdrawal results in severe dermatoses (skin disease without inflammation), marked insomnia, irritability, hyperactivity, and personality changes.

Drug Half-Life: 7–33 hours.

Effexor (brand) ~ Venlafaxine (generic)

Common Usage: SSRI antidepressant; treatment of major depression.

Common dosage: 75–375 mg per day. Most common dosage: 75 mg, three times daily with food.

Major Side Effects: Sleepiness, dry mouth, dizziness, nervousness, upset stomach, constipation, weakness or tiredness, nausea, vomiting, constipation, loss of appetite, weight loss, sweating, sleep disturbances, *increase in blood pressure,* tremor, blurred vision, sexual dysfunction, impotence, chills.

Interactions With Other Medications: Do not take with alcohol. Antihistamines and decongestants may add to side effects. In some patients Cimetadine (Tagamet) may cause more of Effexor to enter the blood stream than is normal. Patients taking routine blood pressure medication

184 / Break Your Prescribed Addiction

need to monitor their blood pressure regularly, especially on higher doses of Effexor. Effexor should not be taken with other similar drugs—SSRIs (Prozac, Paxil, Zoloft) or any other antidepressant medications.

Withdrawal: Terminate by gradually withdrawing Effexor over a period of at least two weeks. Care must be taken that depression does not return after discontinuation of medication. Seek professional help if depression returns. Abrupt withdrawal may include: nervousness, dizziness, insomnia, somnolence, nausea, flu-like syndrome without fever, loss of appetite, nausea, vomiting, upset stomach, sweating, anxiety, agitation, irritability, rapid heart beat, tension headache, neckache, chills, malaise, runny nose, somnolence, excessive dreaming, nightmares, vertigo (dizziness) often with vomiting, visual distortions, and migraine-like headache. The higher the dosage of Effexor the more likelihood of withdrawal symptoms increases with abrupt withdrawal.

Drug Half-Life: 5–7 hours.

Elavil, Endep, Emitrip, Amitril (brand) ~ Amitriptyline (generic)

Common Usage: Tricyclic antidepressant.

Action: Increases the amount of norepinephrine and serotonin in brain neurons. Onset of actions is 2 to 3 weeks.

Common Dosage: 50–100 mg, divided.

Major Side Effects: Dizziness, drowsiness, dry mouth, excessive sweating, fatigue, weight gain/loss, photosensitivity, constipation, diarrhea, vomiting, heart attack, strokes, heart arrhythmias, coma, seizures, incoordination, tremors, paralytic ileus, fever, urinary retention, skin rash, swelling of face and tongue, loss of appetite,

Interactions with Other Medications: Alcohol and

other CNS depressants, narcotics, stimulants, anticholinergic (such as atropine) and anticoagulants increased the effects of amitriptyline. Do not mix with MAOs. Administration of epinephrine or norepinephrine may increase blood pressure. Megadoses of ascorbic acid (Vitamin C) as well as heavy tobacco use may decrease the effectiveness of amitriptyline.

Withdrawal: After prolonged administration, abrupt cessation may produce nausea, headache, malaise, and dizziness. Reducing the dosage gradually within 2 weeks may produce transient symptoms including irritability, restlessness, and dream/sleep disturbances. Rare reports of mania and hypomania have occurred within 2 to 7 days following withdrawal of tricyclic antidepressants.

Drug Half-Life: 10–50 hours.

Flexeril (brand) ~ Cyclobenzaprine (generic)

Common Usage: Muscle relaxant for acute, painful musculoskeletal conditions.

Action: Works within the central nervous system (CNS). Flexeril is structurally related to tricyclic antidepressants and is believed to affect norepinephrine, and acetylcholine.

Common Dosage: 10 mg, three times a day to a maximum of 60 mg per day. Not recommended for more than two to three weeks.

Major Side Effects: Drowsiness, dry mouth, and dizziness. **Less common:** Malaise, tachycardia, arrhythmia, vomiting, diarrhea, gastrointestinal pain, thirst, flatulence, edema of the tongue, abnormal liver function, vertigo, insomnia, depressed mood, anxiety, agitation, abnormal thinking and dreaming, sweating, chest pain, bone marrow suppression.

Contraindications: Hypersensitivity to the drug. Acute

recovery phase of myocardial infarction, and patients with arrhythmias, heart block or conduction disturbances, or congestive heart failure.

Precautions: Should be used with caution in patients with a history of urinary retention, angle-closure glaucoma, increased intraocular pressure, and in patients taking anticholinergic medications.

Precautions: Should not be used if patient is taking a tricyclic antidepressant such as amitriptyline, imipramine or if patient is currently taking or has stopped taking MAO inhibitors within the past two weeks.

Withdrawal: Abrupt withdrawal may cause nausea, headache, and malaise. These are not indicative of addiction.

Drug Half-Life: 1–3 days.

Geodon (brand) ~ Ziprasodone (generic)

Common Usage: Atypical antipsychotic; treatment of schizophrenia and acute mania.

Action: Exact mechanism is unknown, but believed to inhibit synaptic reupake of serotonin and norepineprhine and effects dopamine and histamine levels.

Common Dosage: 20 mg, twice per day.

Major Side Effects: Rash, cognitive and motor impairment, postural hypotension, somnolence, hypertension, vomiting, rhinitis (runny nose), "cold" symptoms, nausea, dyspepsia, diarrhea, dry mouth, dizziness, hypertonia, akathisia, fungal dermatitis, and abnormal vision.

Precautions: Reports of hyperglycemia and/or diabetes development (with ketoacidosis, coma, and deaths), tardive dyskinesia, neurologic malignant syndrome with Geodon use.

Interactions with Other Medications: Decreased plasma levels of ziprasidone when taken with carbamazedine (35%) while increased levels with concurrent ketoconazole (35-45%).

Withdrawal: None listed, but always withdraw slowly. Check with your pharmacist.
Drug Half-Life: 2–5 hours.

Halcion (brand) ~ Triazolam (generic)

Common Usage: Insomnia (not > 6 weeks), sedative-hypnotic, benzodiazepine.
Action: Depresses CNS, especially limbic system, hypothalamus, and thalamus. A calming effect may be seen as triazolam enhances GABA.
Common Dosage: 0.25 mg.
Major Side Effects: Residual drowsiness, dizziness, headache, nervousness, depression, visual disturbances, rapid heart rate > 100, nausea/vomiting, constipation, diarrhea.
Interactions with Other Medications: Other CNS depressants (alcohol, barbiturates, narcotics), anticonvulsants, antihistamines with triazolam potentiates CNS depression. The length of action of triazolam increases with Cimetidine and disulfiram (Antabuse). Caffeine and smoking decreases the effects of triazolam.
Withdrawal: Abrupt withdrawal symptoms include convulsions, tremor, abdominal and muscle cramping/pain, seating, vomiting, depression, restlessness, insomnia. A tapered withdrawal over two weeks to a month is the best method to withdraw the drug.
Drug Half-Life: 1.5–5.5 hours.

Haldol (brand) ~ Haloperidol (generic)

Common Usage: Psychosis, severe anxiety, control of tics and Tourette's syndrome.
Action: Action not clearly established but thought to inhibit reuptake of dopamine in brain synapses.
Common Dosage: 0.5–2 mg daily, divided.

Major Side Effects: Drowsiness, dry mouth, urinary retention, extrapyramidal symptoms—rigidity, motor restlessness, low blood pressure, and tremors, skin eruptions, loss of appetite, diarrhea, nausea/vomiting, blurred vision, tardive dyskinesia (syndrome of potentially irreversible, involuntary slow movements in patients treated with neuroleptic drugs—bizarre tongue and facial stiff neck, difficulty swallowing), neuroleptic malignant syndrome (potentially fatal syndrome with symptoms of heat stroke, fever >106°, muscle rigidity, stupor, profuse sweating, difficulty breathing, incontinence, unstable blood pressure, and arrhythmias).

Interactions with Other Medications: Alcohol and other CNS depressants increases the effect of haloperidol. The addition of lithium in high dosages may produce lethargy and confusion. If methyldopa (Aldomet) is added, symptoms of dementia may result.

Withdrawal: After short-term usage, generally no problems are seen with abrupt withdrawal. After long-term administration, abrupt withdrawal may produce symptoms such as gastritis, nausea, vomiting, dizziness, headache, insomnia, pulse > 100, tremors, extrapyramidal symptoms, neuroleptic malignant syndrome (potentially fatal syndrome with symptoms of fever, muscle rigidity, stupor, profuse sweating, difficulty breathing, incontinence, unstable blood pressure, and arrhythmias).

Drug Half-Life: 21 hours.

Imitrex (brand) ~ Sumatriptan (generic)

Common Usage: Acute migraine headaches.

Action: Selective 5-hydroxytryptamine receptors and vasoconstrictor of the surface arteries of the brain. There is no effect on cerebral (brain) blood flow.

Common Dosage: 3–6 mg subcutaneously and repeat after 1 hour if needed up to 12 mg daily; 20 mg per nasal spray administered 15 minutes apart; 1-2 mg diluted with NS and given over 10 minutes (slow) I.V.

Major Side Effects: Overstimulation, anxiety, hypertension, angina, arrhythmias, peripheral vasoconstriction, palpitations, difficulty breathing, bronchospasm, dizziness, malaise, drowsiness, weakness, bad taste, visual disturbances.

Interactions with Other Medications: Sumatriptan in combination with the cholesterol drug Questran may produce a sore tongue.

Withdrawal: Usually none with short-term use.

Drug Half-Life: 1.5–2.5 hours.

Inderal (brand) ~ Propranolol (generic)

Common Usage: Antihypertensive, antiangina, cardiac arrhythmias, migraine headaches, schizophrenia, tremors due to Parkinson's, aggressive behavior, situational anxiety, acute panic attacks, anxiety.

Action: Blocks certain actions of the sympathetic nervous system such as lowering blood pressure, decreasing oxygen demands of the heart, preventing vasodilation of the cerebral arteries (useful with migraine headaches), and lowering anxiety.

Common Dosage: For cardiac arrhythmias 10–30 mg, three to four times daily; for hypertension, 160–480 mg daily, divided into three or four dosages daily; for angina, 10–20 mg three to four times daily or 80 mg once daily; for prevention of migraine headaches, 160–240 mg daily; for schizophrenia, anxiety 80–1920 mg per day; for tardive dyskinesia, 30–80 mg per day; for acute panic disorders, 40–360 mg per day; for essential tremors, 120–320 mg daily.

Major Side Effects: Dizziness, fatigue, insomnia, weakness, pulse < 60, cold extremities, paresthesia of hands, hypotension (low blood pressure), nausea, diarrhea, depression, severe dizziness, nervousness, lethargy, sedation, diminished concentration, memory loss, congestion heart failure, arrhythmias, palpitations, rash, sweating, dry skin, hyperglycemia (high blood glucose), hypoglycemia (low blood sugar), stomach pain, flatulence, bloating, constipation, dry mouth, loss of appetite, abdominal cramping, mesentery and renal artery thrombosis (clotting), impotence, decreased libido, urinary frequency, eye discomfort, vision, disturbances, anxiety, bizarre dreams, change in behavior, wheezing, nasal stuffiness, runny nose, sore throat, joint and back pains.

Interactions with Other Medications: Aluminum hydroxide greatly reduce intestinal absorption. Alcohol slows the rate of absorption whereas phenytoin, phenobarbitone, and rifampin accelerate Inderal's clearance. When used concomitantly with chlorpromazine, it results in increased plasma levels of both drugs. Antipyrine and lidocaine, and theophylline have reduced clearances, if used concomitantly with Inderal. Cimetidine decrease liver metabolism of propranolol delaying elimination and increasing blood levels. Lower T_3 may result if used concurrently.

Withdrawal: Abrupt withdrawal symptoms include sweating, severe headache, tremors, malaise, palpitation, rebound hypertension, heat attack, life-threatening arrhythmias in angina patients, hyperthyroidism. After long-term administration especially in patients with heart disease, gradual reduction over 1 to 2 weeks with monitoring of patients is preferred.

Drug Half-Life: 3.4–6 hours after repeat dosing.

Klonopin (brand) ~ Clonazapam (generic)

Common Usage: Anticonvulsant—seizure control. (Benziodiazepine derivative). Other applications include: anxiety, phobia, panic disorder, tardive dyskinesia, insomnia.

Action: Not completely understood. CNS depression, and may increase effects of GABA (inhibitory neurotransmitter) in the brain. Clonazapam is capable of suppressing the spike and wave discharge in a absence seizures while decreasing the frequency, amplitude, duration, and spread offf motor seizures.

Common Dosage: 0.75–1.5 mg per day, divided, to a maximum of 20 mg per day in adults.

Major Side Effects: Drowsiness, ataxia (unsteady gait), abnormal eye movement, behavior problems, dizziness, confusion, headache, insomnia, lethargy, amnesia, hallucinations, chest congestion, palpitations, loss of appetite, nausea, vomiting, constipation, diarrhea, increased salivation, dry mouth, increased appetite, skin rashes, tremor, abnormal blood tests.

Interactions with Other Medications: Alcohol, barbiturates, narcotics, hypnotics, antianxiety, phenothiazines, antipsychotics, antidepressants, anticonvulsants, and antihistamines enhance clonazepam's effect. Carbamazepine, phenytoin (Dilantin), phenobarbital decrease the effectiveness of clonazapam.

Withdrawal: Clonazapam should never be discontinued abruptly. Abrupt withdrawal may produce convulsions, psychosis, hallucinations, anxiety, trembling, seizures, vision problems, nightmares, difficulty sleeping, malaise, dizziness, abdominal and muscle cramps, exaggerated feeling of depression and unrest.

Drug Half-Life: 18–50 hours.

Lexapro (brand) ~ Escitalopram (generic)

Common Usage: Antidepressant used to treat major depressive disorder and Generalized Anxiety Disorder (GAD).

Action: Selective serotonin reuptake inhibitor (SSRI).

Common Dosage: 10 mg, once daily.

Major Side Effects: Insomnia, ejaculation disorder (primarily ejaculatory delay), nausea, increased sweating, fatigue, and somnolence, are the most common side effects occurring in approximately 5% of patients. Other frequent side effects include dry mouth, dizziness, diarrhea, constipation, flu-like symptoms, decreased appetite, decreased libido, rhinitis, and impotence.

Contraindications: Do not use with MAO inhibitors or within 14 days of discontinuing an MAO. Do not use with Celexa (brand) or citalopram (generic).

Precautions: Abnormal bleeding potential— epidemiological studies have demonstrated an association between use of psychotropic drugs that interfere with serotonin reuptake and the occurrence of upper gastrointestinal (GI) bleeding. Taking nonsteroidal anti-inflammatory drugs (NSAID) or aspirin increases the risk of GI bleeding. Increased potential for suicide, and activation of mania in some patients.

Pregnancy: Neonates exposed to Lexapro and other SSRIs or SNRI, late in the third trimester, have developed complications requiring prolonged hospitalization, respiratory support, and tube feeding.

Withdrawal: Do not withdraw drug suddenly. There have been reports of adverse events occurring upon discontinuation of Lexapro as well as other SSRI drugs, particularly when abrupt, including the following: dysphoric mood, irritability, agitation, dizziness, sensory disturbances (e.g., paresthesias such as electric shock sensations), anxiety, confusion, headache, lethargy, emotional lability, insomnia, and hypomania.

Drug Half-Life: 27–34 hours. Half-life increases with patients over 65 years, or impaired liver and kidney function.

Lorcet (brand) ~ Hydrocodone (generic)

Common Usage: Moderate to moderately severe pain.

Action: Exact mechanism is unknown, but believed to attach to opiate receptors in brain.

Common Dosage: 1 tablet every 4 to 6 hours; not to exceed 6 tablets per day.

Major Side Effects: Drowsiness, dizziness, light-headedness, nausea, vomiting, mental clouding, lethargy, impairment of mental and physical performance, anxiety, fear, mood changes, physical and mental dependence.

Interactions with Other Medications: Alcohol, antianxiety, antipsychotic, narcotic analgesics may potentiate CNS depression.

Withdrawal: After administration as short as a month, withdrawal symptoms may occur with abrupt withdrawal. Symptoms may occur after the drug is withheld 4–12 hours. Symptoms include craving for the drug, insomnia, yawning, nausea, vomiting, sweating, tremors, diarrhea, mental depression, abdominal and muscle cramping/ aches, chills, and anxiety.

Drug Half-Life: 0.9–3.25 hours.

Ludiomil (brand) ~ Maprotiline (generic)

Common Usage: Tetracyclic Antidepressant; depression with depressive anxiety and manic-depressive illness.

Action: Exact mechanism is unknown, but blocks reuptake of norepinephrine increasing the concentration in the brain synapses.

Common Dosage: 150–225 mg per day

Major Side Effects: Drowsiness, dizziness, tremor, dry mouth, constipation, nervousness, anxiety, insomnia, headache, agitation, blurred vision, fatigue, nausea, altered liver function tests, jaundice, and seizures.

Interactions with Other Medications: The addition of MAOs may cause a hypertensive and/or hyperpyretic crisis. Increased blood pressure may be seen with the addition of amphetamines. Alcohol, barbiturates, and cimetidine potentiate effects of maprotiline. Increased blood levels of maprotiline may be seen with the addition of methylphenidate (Ritalin), phenothiazines (Thorazine), or cimetidine, increased blood levels may produce seizures. Smoking increases the metabolism of maprotiline.

Withdrawal: Abrupt withdrawal may cause flu-like symptoms without fever, anxiety, agitation, irritability, cold sweats, rapid pulse >100, tension headaches, neck pain, insomnia, sleepiness, excessive dreaming /nightmares. Withdrawal symptoms usually begin 2 to 4 days (up to 7) after acute withdrawal of maprotiline. The withdrawal symptoms may last for 1 to 2 weeks, and are not life threatening. Gradual withdrawal should minimize withdrawal symptoms. Titration over at least 2 weeks to a month is always the preferred method.

Drug Half-Life: 27–58 hours.

Luvox (brand) ~ Fluvoxamine (generic)

Common Use: SSRI, treatment of obsessive-compulsive disorder.

Action: Mechanism of action is believed to be specific serotonin reuptake inhibition of brain neurons.

Common Dosage: 100–300 mg per day.

Major Side Effects: Unlike the other SSRI antidepressants, Luvox has a tendency to make patients drowsy, and therefore, is often given at bedtime. Other side effects include somnolence, nervousness, anxiety, dizziness, shakiness, agitation, feeling of general weakness, nausea, vomiting and upset stomach, lack of appetite, diarrhea, headache, asthenia (loss of muscle strength or weakness), tremor, sexual dysfunction, dry mouth and sweating.

Interactions With Other Medications: Do not take with alcohol. Products or foods containing tryptophan (poultry, pork, and powdered protein drink mixes are among the highest) and 5-HTP are not recommended. They may cause severe headache, nausea, sweating and dizziness. This same reaction can occur with tramadol (Ultram), fenfluramine (Pondimen) and dexfenfluramine (ReDux). Decongestants and antihistamines may exacerbate the severity of certain side effects, impairing judgment while driving. Dextromethoraphan ("DM" in many over-the-counter and prescription cough preparations) and codeine can cause hallucinations in patients taking SSRIs. There may be a possibility of an interaction with sumitriptan (Imitrex). Patients already on drugs such as propanolol (Inderal) and other beta blockers, metoprolol (Lopressor), carbamazepine (Tegretol), clozapine (Clozaril), diltiazem (Cardizem), lithium, methadone, theophylline (Theo-Dur, Slo-BID) and warfarin (Coumadin), should be monitored closely to make adjustments (usually a decrease) to the usual doses of these drugs since starting Luvox.

Withdrawal: Abrupt cessation may produce headaches, weakness, nausea, vomiting, insomnia, sleepiness, nervousness, agitation, dizziness, anxiety, anorexia, dry mouth, abdominal pain, and upset stomach.

Half Life: 15.6 hours.

Mellaril (brand) ~ Thioridazine (generic)

Common Usage: Antipsychotic, severe behavioral problems such as combativeness and/or explosive hyperexcitable behavior in children, and mild to moderate depression with variable degrees of anxiety.

Action: Exact mechanism is not fully understood. It is believed to block postsynaptic dopamine receptors in basal ganglia, limbic system, hypothalamus, brain stem,

and medulla. Thioridazine inhibits dopamine neurotransmission at the synapses, and blocks transmission of other
amines (such as GABA) or neurotransmitters.

Common Dosage: 200–800 mg per day, divided.

Major Side Effects: Tardive dyskinesia (syndrome of
potentially irreversible, involuntary slow movements in
patients treated with neuroleptic drugs—bizarre tongue
and facial movements, stiff neck, difficulty swallowing),
drowsiness, headache, dry mouth, constipation, urinary
retention (especially in men with benign prostatic hyper-
tropy), dizziness upon standing, heart arrhythmias, rash,
lack of appetite, retinopathy (impaired vision), weight
gain, extrapyramidal symptoms such as rigidity, motor
restlessness and tremor, sun sensitivity, neuroleptic malignant syndrome (potentially fatal syndrome with symptoms of fever, muscle rigidity, stupor, profuse sweating,
difficulty breathing, incontinence, unstable blood pressure, and arrhythmias), abnormal blood tests, jaundice,
turns urine pink to reddish-brown in color.

Interactions with Other Medications: Caution should
be utilized when thioridazine is combined with CNS depressants such as alcohol, narcotics, barbiturates, anticholinergic (atropine) drugs as their effects are increased.
Antacids and magnesium reduce absorption of thioridazine. If propanolol (Inderal) is added to thioridazine, both
drugs have increased plasma levels. If combined with phenytoin (Dilantin), increased levels of phenytoin and risk
of toxicity. Drinks containing caffeine such as colas, teas,
or coffee counteract antipsychotic effect. Dairy products
cause the drug to remain in the body longer.

Withdrawal: If abruptly stopped after long-term use or
high dose therapy, withdrawal symptoms include headaches, nausea, dizziness, and increased heart rate. Symptoms usually begin 2 to 4 days and last for as much as 2

weeks. Gradual withdrawal over 2 weeks to a month will decrease withdrawal symptoms. The psychosis, depression, or behavioral problems may return after discontinuation of the medication.

Drug Half-Life: 9–30 hours.

Meridia (brand) ~ Sibutramine (generic)

Common Usage: Appetite suppressant, weight loss for obese (at least 20% over ideal body weight) in combination with monitored diet treatment plan that includes diet, exercise, and behavior changes.

Action: Norephinephrine, serotonin, and dopamine reuptake prolonging the brain's appetite regulating neurotransmitters.

Common Dosage: 10–15 mg once daily.

Major Side Effects: Headache, increasing blood pressure, loss of appetite, increased appetite, backache, constipation, dry mouth, insomnia, dizziness, flu-like symptoms, runny nose, sore throat, nervousness, inflammation/infection of sinuses, rash, nausea, upset stomach, injury/accident, joint pains, abdominal pain, and loss of strength. Other centrally acting weight loss drugs that cause a release of serotonin have been connected with pulmonary hypertension. Certain Rat studies demonstrated damage to serotonin network, but it is unknown if this happens in humans.

Interactions with Other Medications: Alcohol may increase sedative effects. Certain cold/allergy medications that contain phenylpropanolamine, ephedrine, or pseudoephedrine may cause increase in blood pressure. Combining sibutramine with other SSRI antidepressants, any drug that alters serotonin activity or Imitrex (sumatriptan succinate), certain pain medications such as

Demerol, Fontanel, and Talwin may cause serious, sometimes fatal reactions such as serotonin syndrome. Do not combine with tryptophan or 5-HTP or foods containing these. Caution should be utilized because of interactions if sibutamine is combined with ketoconazole, (Nizoral), phenytoin (Dilantin), warfarin (Coumadin), erythromycin (E-Mycin), cimetidine Tagamet, lithium (Eskalith).

Withdrawal: Discontinuation of sibutamine produced no side effects with abrupt withdrawal.

Drug Half Life: 14–16 hours.

Neurontin (brand) ~ Gabapentin (generic)

Common Usage: Analgesic, anticonvulsant, and antiseizure.

Action: Exact method of action is unknown. Gabapentin is structurally related to the neurotransmitter GABA (Gamma Amino Butyric Acid), but it does not modify GABA, it is not converted metabolically into GABA or a GABA agonist, and it is not an inhibitor of GABA uptake or degradation. In vitro studies have revealed a gabapentin binding site in areas of the rat's brain including neocortex and hippocampus.

Common Dosage: 1800–3600 mg daily. No benefit of treatment was seen between the 1800 and the 3600 mg dose.

Major Side Effects: May cause dizziness, somnolence and other signs of central nervous system depression, asthenia, diarrhea, dry mouth, peripheral edema, fatigue, viral infection, headache, anorexia, flatulence, gingivitis, paresthesias, and anxiety.

Interactions with Other Medications: Decreased clearance of gabapentin and alteration of renal function occurs when used with cimetidine. Maalox reduces Gabapentin levels by 25% if taken within 2 hours of Maalox ingestion.

Precautions: In rat studies gabapentin induced pancreatic carcinogenesis. It is not known whether gabapentin has the ability to increase cell proliferation in other cell types or in other species, including humans.

Withdrawal: Do not stop drug suddenly especially when being used in the treatment of epilepsy.

Drug Half-Life: 5–7 hours.

Norgesic Forte (brand) ~ Orphenadrine (generic)

Common Usage: Muscle relaxant.

Action: Central nervous system (CNS), anticholinergic.

Common Dosage: ½ to 1 tablet every 4 to 6 hours (50 mg to a maximum 400 mg daily).

Major Side Effects: Tachycardia, transient dizziness or syncope, GI bleeding or upset, dry mouth, blurred vision, weakness, headache, increased intraocular pressure, urinary retention, rash, blood dyscrasias.

Interactions with Other Medications: Alcohol, aspirin, NSAIDS, corticosteroids and anticoagulants increase risk of GI bleeding or ulceration. Oral hypoglycemics and anticholinergics potentiated. Protein bound drugs (e.g. warfarin) may be displaced. Antagonizes steroids, barbiturates, phenylbutazone and uricosurics. Proproxphene may cause tremor and mental confusion.

Contraindications: NSAID allergy, varicella or influenza in teenagers, glaucoma, achalasia, prostatic hypertrophy, bladder neck or GI obstruction, myasthenia gravis.

Precautions: Coronary disease, insufficiency or tachycardia, history of bronchospasm, peptic ulcer, and coagulation disorders. Monitor blood pressure, BUN, uric acid levels.

Withdrawal: No specfic information available; check with your pharmacist.

Drug Half-Life: No information.

Norpramin (brand) ~ Desipramine (generic)

Common Usage: Tricyclic antidepressant—major depression and Attention Deficit Hyperactivity Disorder.
Action: selective norepinephrine reuptake inhibitor (SNRI).
Common Dosage: 150–250 mg at bedtime.
Major Side Effects: Dry mouth, constipation, blurred vision, sedation, weight gain, sexual dysfunction, orthostatic hypotension, pro-arrhythmic effects, and sinus tachycardia.
Drug Interactions: Do not take with Clonidine, Class I antiarrhythmics (e.g. Quinidine, Flecainide), coumadin, aspirin, or fluoxetine (Prozac, Sarafem).
Precautions: Overdose causes cardiotoxicity and death.
Withdrawal: Abrupt withdrawal symptoms following long-term administration include nausea, severe dizziness, malaise, insomnia, and nightmares.
Drug Half-Life: 21 hours.

Oxycontin (Brand) ~ Oxycodone (generic)

Common Usage: Analgesic; schedule II controlled substance with an abuse liability similar to morphine.
Action: Opioid agonist.
Common Dosage: Must be individualized, it is supplied in 10, 20, 40, 80 and 160 mg tablets. 80 mg and 160 mg tablets should only be used in opioid-tolerant patients.
Major Side Effects: Respiratory depression, reduction in stomach and bowel motility, altered mental state, nausea, vomiting, may cause itching, flushing, red eyes, sweating, and orthostatic hypotension.
Drug Interactions: The route of elimination may be blocked when taken with certain cardiovascular drugs including amiodarone and quinidine as well as polycyclic antidepressants.
Precautions: Hepatic (liver) impairment.

Withdrawal: Doses should be tapered gradually to prevent signs and symptoms of withdrawal in the physically dependent patient.
Drug Half-Life: 4.5 hours

Pamelor (brand) ~ Nortriptyline (generic)

Common Usage: Tricyclic antidepressant—major depression with lack of interest; bipolar depression.
Action: Blocks reuptake of norepinephrine and serotonin at synapse in brain, increasing the concentration of these neurotransmitters.
Common Dosage: 25 mg, three or four times daily.
Major Side Effects: Drowsiness, dizziness, dry mouth, excessive sweating, weight gain, weakness, low blood pressure upon standing, pulse > 100, EKG changes, constipation, urinary retention, headache, fatigue, confusion, lethargy, memory defects, nausea/vomiting, loss of appetite, nasal congestion.
Interactions with Other Medications: Concurrent use of MAOs will result in hypertensive and hyperpyretic (fever > 106°F.) crisis, rapid heartbeats > 100, severe seizures, and death. Amphetamines enhance cardiac and hypertensive effects of these drugs. Increased nortriptyline levels result with the addition of cimetidine, methylphenidate, phenothiazines, or haloperidol. Alcohol, barbiturates, benzodiazepines and other CNS depressants will increase CNS effect if added to nortriptyline. Clonidine decreases effects nortriptyline. Smoking will increase nortriptyline metabolism.
Withdrawal: Abrupt withdrawal after long-term therapy may produce nausea, headache, severe dizziness, malaise, insomnia, and nightmares. The gradual withdrawal utilizing a taper technique over at least 2 weeks to a month is

best. After discontinuing any antidepressant medication, depression may return. Allow at least two weeks after discontinuing before adding any other medication to allow the medication to clear the body totally.
Drug Half-Life: 16–90 hours.

Parnate (brand) ~Tranylcypromine(generic)

Common Usage: MAO—major depressive episodes.
Action: Monoamine oxidase inhibitor. Increases the concentration of epinephrine, norepinephrine, and serotonin in storage sites throughout the nervous system.
Common Dosage: 30 mg daily in divided doses.
Major Side Effects: Orthostatic hypotension, hypertensive crises, headache, CNS overstimulation, seizures, changes in blood sugar, drowsiness, dry mouth, GI disturbances, tachycardia, anorexia, impotence, rash, hepatitis, edema.
Drug Interactions: Hypertensive crises with sympathomimetics, levodopa, and high-tyramine foods (including cheese, salami, chocolate, wine, beer, pickled herring, chicken livers, yeast extract, yogurt, broad beans, others). Caution with antidiabetic agents, antiparkinson agents, disulfiram. Potentiates CNS depressants, antihypertensives. Psychosis with dextromethrophan. Circulatory collapse, coma, death with meperidine. Do not start within 5 weeks of fluoxetine (Prozac), or 2 weeks of sertraline (Zoloft), paroxetine (Paxil), bupropion (Wellbutrin) or citalopram (Celexa), or one week of venlafaxine (Effexor).
Contraindications: Pheochromocytoma (tumor of the adrenal gland), cardiovascular, cerebrovascular, or liver disease, hypertension, chronic headache. To avoid potentially severe or fatal interactions, allow sufficient drug-free interval between tranylcypromine and: amphetamines, pseudoephedrine, tricyclic antidepressants, SSRIs or other

neurotransmitter reuptake inhibitors, CNS depressants (e.g. alcohol, barbiturates, narcotics), antihistamines, antihypertensives, anesthetics, bupropion (Wellbutrin), buspirone, carbamazepine, cyclobenzaprine, dibenzazepines, diuretics, dextromethorphan, dopamine, other MAOIs (e.g. phenelzine, selegiline, furazolidone, isocarboxazid), levadopa, methyldopa, methylphenidate, tryptophan, phenylalanine, or tyramine-containing foods, excess caffeine or chocolate.

Precautions: Hypotension, suicidal tendencies, psychosis, epilepsy, hyperthyroidism, and surgery. There have been reports of drug dependency occurring with patients using more than the therapeutic dose.

Withdrawal: Avoid abrupt cessation.

Drug Half-Life: 24 hours.

Other MAOs:

Furoxone (brand) ~ Furazolidone (generic)

Marplan (brand) ~ Isocarboxazid (generic)

Eutony (brand) ~ Pargyline (generic)

Procarbazine (brand) ~ Phenelzine (generic)

Paxil (brand) ~ Paroxetine (generic)

Common Usage: Antidepressant; treatment of major depression, panic disorder, and obsessive-compulsive disorder.

Action: Potentiates serotonin activity in CNS from inhibition of neuronal reuptake of serotonin.

Common Dosages: 10 to 50 mg per day maximum. In the elderly or patients with liver or kidney disease, the dosage should not exceed 40 mg per day.

Major Side Effects:: The most common side effects include a generalized feeling of weakness, sedation, headaches, nervousness, shakiness, nausea, upset stomach, dizziness, light-headedness, dry mouth, constipation, or diarrhea, sweating, decrease in appetite, drowsiness, insomnia, anxiety and sexual disturbance (male more than female).

Interactions With Other Medications: Do not take with alcohol. Products or foods containing tryptophan or 5-HTP are not recommended as they may cause severe headaches, nausea, sweating, and dizziness. Certain drugs used in the treatment of Parkinson's disease (Sinemet, Levadopa) may be rendered less effective when risperidone is added to current drug therapy. Carbamazepine (Tegretol) may interfere with resperidone's effectiveness by clearing risperidone from the body too quickly. Clozapine (Clozaril), another psychotropic drug, may increase the effect of risperidone by slowing down the rate at which risperidone clears from the body. Certain over-the-counter medications such as antihistamines found in cough and cold remedies may have an additive effect on the severity of some side effects.

Withdrawal: Stop over a period of at least two weeks to several months by slowly reducing dosage. Monitor to make sure depression does not return after discontinuation of medication. Seek professional help if depression returns. Abrupt withdrawal may include: nervousness, dizziness, insomnia, somnolence, nausea, flu-like syndrome without fever, loss of appetite, nausea, vomiting, upset stomach, sweating, anxiety, agitation, irritability, rapid heart beat, tension headache, neck aches, chills, malaise, runny nose, somnolence, excessive dreaming, nightmares, vertigo (dizziness) often with vomiting, visual distortions, migraine-like headache, and electric shock-like sensations. The higher the dosage of Paxil, the more the likelihood withdrawal symptoms will increase

with abrupt withdrawal.
Drug Half-Life: 15.6 hours.

Prozac (brand) ~ Fluoxetine (generic)

Common Use: SSRI; treatment of obsessive-compulsive disorder.
Action: Serotonin reuptake in brain neurons.
Common Dosage: 20–80 mg per day.
Major Side Effects: This drug must not be discontinued suddenly (without physician's guidance) as depression may return quickly and more severely than when the drug was first started. Headache, nervousness, sleeplessness, drowsiness, anxiety, shakiness, dizziness, rash, agitation, general feeling of weakness or fatigue, nausea and upset stomach (take with food or milk), diarrhea, decreased appetite, constipation, and decreased sexual desire (male & female), hostility, akathisia. Some side effects may lessen in severity or even subside within a few weeks of therapy. *The Journal of Clinical Psychiatry,* September 1989, reported that Prozac caused akathisia or drug induced insanity in 10 to 25% of patients. Symptoms of akathisia include hallucinations, aggression, self-destructive outbursts, terror, anger, hostility, hatred, and rage.
Interactions With Other Medications: Not to be taken with alcohol. Products or foods containing tryptophan (i.e., poultry, veal, some health store protein powders) or 5-HTP are not recommended. They may cause agitation, restlessness, severe headache, nausea, gastrointestinal distress, sweating and dizziness. Patients currently taking carbamazepine (Tegretol), lithium, warfarin (Coumadin), phenytoin (Dilantin) and cimetadine (Tagamet) may need to have the dosages of these drugs adjusted by their physician after Prozac is added to the regimen. Over-the-counter drugs

such as decongestants and antihistamines may increase the severity of certain side effects. There may be a possibility of an interaction with sumatriptan (Imitrex), however, available studies have not produced consistent results. There have been reports that patients taking buspirone (Buspar), especially for OCD, have had a worsening of their condition when Prozac was added.

Withdrawal Effects: Abrupt withdrawal may cause severe withdrawal reactions including *crashing* into depression with suicidal or violent behavior. According to the manufacturer, Eli Lilly, Fluoxetine may be terminated by simply discontinuing the drug.

Half-Life: 2–3 days drug and 7–9 days active components. Drug is seen for several weeks in plasma.

Remeron (brand) ~ Mirtazapine (generic)

Common Usage: Antidepressant—treatment of major depression.

Action: Unknown but suggests to effect central adrenergic and serotonergic activity.

Common Dosage: 15-45 mg per day at bedtime.

Major Side Effects: Sedation, drowsiness, increased appetite/weight gain, dizziness, dry mouth, constipation, flu-like symptoms, headache, blurred vision, hypertension (increased blood pressure), nausea/vomiting, thirst, muscle and joint pains, apathy, agitation, anxiety, depression, amnesia, twitching, increased cough, inflammation of sinuses, rash, urinary tract infection.

Interactions with Other Medications: Alcohol, benzodiazepines (Valium, Xanax, Ativan, etc.), antihistamines, and prescription painkillers may increase Mirtazapine's effect, impairing cognitive, motor, and driving skills. The addition of CNS stimulants such as phentermine (Fastin),

dextroamphetamine (Dexedrine), or methylphenidate (Ritalin) may produce an increase in agitation or even mania in bipolar patients.
Withdrawal: Withdraw slowly. Do not abruptly stop.
Drug Half-Life: 20–40 hours.

Restoril (brand) ~ Temazepam (generic)

Common Usage: Sedative-hypnotic; benzodiazepine; Short-term insomnia (generally 7-10 days).
Action: Depression of CNS and limbic system. It is believed to potentiate the effects of GABA in the brain, thereby producing a calming effect.
Common Dosage: 7.5–15 mg at bedtime.
Major Side Effects: Physical and psychological dependence, drowsiness, headache, dizziness, nausea, nervousness, lethargy, fatigue, hangover, palpitations, loss of appetite, diarrhea, anxiety, weakness, blurred vision, dry mouth.
Interaction With Other Medications: Other CNS depressants such as alcohol, barbiturates, narcotics, antihistamines, and anticonvulsants cause additional CNS depression.
Withdrawal: Abrupt withdraw can cause insomnia, aggravated feeling of depression and unrest without cause, convulsions, tremor, abdominal and muscle cramping, vomiting, and sweating. Restoril is best discontinued gradually over 1 to 2 weeks. Depression may return more severely than prior to the drug.
Drug Half-Life: 10–20 hours.

Risperdal (brand) ~ Risperidone (generic)

Common Usage: Atypical antipsychotic.
Action: Unknown.
Common Dosage: 0.5–3 mg, twice daily.

Major Side Effects: Insomnia, agitation, anxiety, aggressive reaction, headache, dizziness, constipation, nausea, vomiting, abdominal pain, coughing, back pain, fever, chest pain, rash, dry skin, drowsiness (which may affect ability to drive), fatigue, sun-sensitivity, and sexual dysfunction.

Interactions With Other Medications: Do not take with alcohol. Certain drugs used in the treatment of Parkinson's disease (Sinemet, Levadopa) may be rendered less effective when risperidone is added to current drug therapy. Carbamazepine (Tegretol) may interfere with risperidone's effectiveness by clearing risperidone from the body too quickly. Clozapine (Clozaril) may increase the effect of risperidone by slowing down the rate at which risperidone clears from the body. Antihistamines and decongestants may have an additive effect on the severity of some side effects.

Withdrawal: Symptoms begin 2 to 4 days (up to 7 days) after stopping risperidone. Withdrawal symptoms can persist for 2 weeks. It is best to gradually withdraw over 1 to 2 weeks. Abrupt withdrawal may generate gastrointestinal upset, nausea, vomiting, diarrhea, headaches, insomnia, nightmares, sweating, runny nose, increased appetite, giddiness, dizziness, cold and warm sensation, tremors, and rapid heart beats.

Precautions: Hyperglycemia and/or diabetes development (with ketoacidosis, coma, and deaths) with risperidone use.

Drug Half-Life: 20 hours.

Ritalin (brand) ~ Methylphenidate (generic)
Focalin (brand) ~ Dexmethylphenidate
Metadate (brand) ~ Methylphenidate (generic)

Common Usage: CNS stimulant; attention deficit disorder, narcolepsy.

Action: Exact mechanism unknown, but believed to activate the brain stem and cortex.

Common Dosage: 10–60 mg per day.

Major Side Effects: Nervousness, insomnia, skin rash, dermatitis, appetite loss, headache, weight loss, rapid heartbeats, nausea, blood pressure and pulse changes, cardiac arrhythmias, palpitations, abdominal pains, and suppressed growth in children.

Interactions with Other Medications: Should not be used in patients with Tourette's syndrome, high blood pressure, heart problems or glaucoma. An increased number, duration, and severity of seizures may be seen with methylphenidate administration. Foods and drinks with caffeine increase methylphenidate's effects. Anticoagulants (Coumadin), anticonvulsants (Dilantin, Phenobarbital) or Primidone (Mysoline), tricyclic antidepressants amitriptyline (Elavil) or imipramine (Tofranil) decrease metabolism and increase activity of methylphenidate. Concurrent administration of methylphenidate with antihypertensive (blood pressure) medications may cause increase blood pressure and heart rate causing a hypertensive crisis. Over the counter cold and allergy medications (Sudafed), phenylephrine, phenylpropanolamine (Dimetapp) may exacerbate side effects such as insomnia and nervousness which may, in turn, elevate blood pressure and heart rate more.

Withdrawal: Sudden discontinuation may produce extreme fatigue, lethargy, increased dreaming, mental depression, and suicidal ideations.

Drug Half Life: 2-4 hours.

Sarafem: See Prozac.

Serax (brand) ~ Oxazepam (generic)

Common Usage: Antianxiety—short-term anxiety, tension; benzodiazepine.

Action: Depresses the CNS at limbic system and reticular formation by increasing inhibitory neurotransmitter, GABA.

Common Dosage: 15–30 mg daily, divided into 3 to 4 dosages.

Major Side Effects: Drowsiness, lethargy, fainting, hangover, nausea, vomiting, abdominal discomfort, lightheadedness, headache, disorientation, confusion, increased appetite, constipation, diarrhea, weight gain/loss, dry mouth, bitter/metallic taste, rash, itchy skin, increased or decreased libido, difficulty in urination, urinary retention, hyper/hypotension, pulse >100 or < 60, palpitations, abnormal blood tests, blurred vision, joint pains, muscle aches, shortness of breath. For the first few weeks after beginning oxazepam paradoxical reactions may occur distinguished by sleep disorders, anxiety, and nervousness.

Interactions with Other Medications: Alcohol, antihistamines, barbiturates, and phenothiazines potentiate CNS depressants leading to drowsiness, lethargy, stupor, respiratory collapse, coma, or death. Tricyclic antidepressants may cause additive sedative effects. Increased effects of benzodiazepines are seen with cimetidine, digoxin, phenytoin, probenecid, propoxyphene, propranolol, ketoconazole, fluoxetine, isoniazid, valproic acid, and erythromycin. Rantidine decreases absorption of benzodiazepines. Theophylline decreases sedative effects of benzodiazepines.

Withdrawal: Abrupt withdrawal after long-term use may produce anxiety, irritability, insomnia, psychotic behavior, convulsions, depression, hallucinations, sweating, vomiting, depression, restlessness, insomnia and severe abdominal and muscle cramps. Tapering the medication over at

least a 2-week to a month decreases withdrawal effects.
Drug Half-Life: 5–20 hours.

Seroquel (brand) ~ Quetiapine (generic)

Common Usage: Atypical antipsychotic; treatment of schizophrenia and acute mania.

Action: Exact mechanism is unknown, but believed to inhibit synaptic reupake of serotonin and norepineprhine and effects dopamine and histamine levels.

Common Dosage: 400–800 mg per day.

Major Side Effects: Cholesterol and triglyceride elevation, somnolence, headache, dry mouth, pain, tachycardia, agitation, dizziness, weight gain, nausea, constipation, uncontrollable movements, cataract development, flu-like symptoms, peripheral edema.

Precautions: Reports of hyperglycemia and/or diabetes development (with ketoacidosis, coma, and deaths), tardive dyskinesia, neurologic malignant syndrome with Seroquel use. Do not use if patient has a history of Q-T prolongation (such as syncope).

Interactions with Other Medications: Decreased plasma levels of quetiapine when taken with dilantin, thioridazine (65%), and cimetidine (20%). With coadministration of Seroquel, decreased levels of lorazepam.

Withdrawal: None listed, but check with your pharmacist.

Drug Half-Life: 6 hours.

Serzone (brand) ~ Nefazodone (generic)

Common Usage: Atypical antidepressant, treatment of major depression.

Action: Nefazodone inhibits neuronal reuptake of serotonin and norepinephrine.

Common Dosage: 200–600 mg per day.

Major Side Effects: Headache, asthenia (weakness), drowsiness, dry mouth, nausea, and upset stomach, constipation, dizziness, insomnia, blurred or abnormal vision, sexual dysfunction, light-headedness, confusion, constipation, infection, eye pain, and postural hypotension (drop in blood pressure when going from a sitting position to a standing position).

Interactions With Other Medications: Do not take with alcohol. Serious and possibly fatal reactions could occur while taking monoamine oxidase inhibitors (MAOIs)—Nardil or Parnate, with nefazodone. Nefazodone should also not be taken with triazolam (Halcion) or alprazolam (Xanax) especially in elderly patients where interaction may cause severe impairment of thinking and movement. Terfenadine (Seldane), astemizole (Hismanal), and cisapride (Propulsid) are also not recommended for use with serzone, due to possibility of negative side effects on the heart. Over the counter decongestants and antihistamines may interfere with the heart.

Withdrawal: Sudden withdrawal of Serzone includes nausea, dizziness, insomnia, asthenia, and agitation.

Drug Half-Life: 4 hours.

Sinequan (brand) ~ Doxepin (generic)

Common Use: Tricyclic antidepressant, chronic pain syndrome, anxiety, diabetic neuropathy.

Action: Serotonin and norepinephrine activity may be increased in descending pain inhibitory pathways. Analgesia effect occurs after 5 days while antidepressant effect takes 1 to 2 weeks.

Common Dosage: 20–50 mg three times daily, or one dose at bedtime. Dosage is titrated upward every 3 to 4 weeks.

Major Side Effects: Arrhythmias, hypertension, respiratory depression, confusion, disorientation, nausea, vomiting, constipation, urinary retention, blurred vision, decreased libido.

Interactions with Other Medications: Increased risk of hyperthermia and paralytic ileus with concomitant administration of anticholinergics such as atropine, phenothiazines, and thyroid medication. Convulsions and death may occur when mixed with MAOs. CNS depressants and alcohol potentiate doxepin.

Toxicity Manifestations: Chronic dream and sleep disturbances, akathisia (constant restlessness), anxiety, chills, headache, dizziness, nausea and vomiting.

Withdrawal: Abrupt withdrawal after long-term use may produce insomnia, disturbed REM sleep, nausea, anxiety, and fatigue.

Half-Life: 8–24 hours.

Soma (brand) ~ Carisoprodol (generic)

Common Usage: Relief of pain, muscle spasm, and limited mobillty associated with acute, painful musculoskeletal conditions.

Action: Centrally acting muscle relaxant.

Common Dosage: 1 or 2 tablets, four times daily.

Major Side Effects: Drowsiness, dizziness, vertigo, ataxia, tremor, agitation, irritability, headache, depressive reactions, and insomnia.

Drug Interactions: Increased clotting times with Coumadin. Enhancement of hypoglycemia may occur with oral antidiabetic drugs. Do not use with alcohol, other CNS depressants, or psychotropic drugs.

Precautions: Impairs mental/physical ability to drive a vehicle or operate machinery.

Withdrawal: In some individuals, abrupt cessation of Soma produces symptoms such as abdominal cramps,

insomnia, chilliness, headache, and nausea. Most people report no withdrawal signs when stopping this drug.
Precautions: Impairs mental/physical ability to drive a vehicle or operate machinery.
Drug Half-Life: 4–6 hours.

Sonata (brand) ~ Zeleplon (generic)

Common Usage: Hypnotic/sedative for short-term treatment of insomnia; Class IV Scheduled controlled substance.
Action: Interacts with the Gamma-Amino Butyric Acid-(GABA) benzodiazepines (GABA-BZ) receptor complex.
Common Dosage: 10–20 mg.
Major Side Effects: Drowsiness, dizziness, lightheadedness, memory impairment and difficulty with coordination.
Drug Interactions: Do not take with alcohol.
Precautions: A variety of abnormal thinking and behavior changes occur with sedative/hypnotics meds including decreased inhibition (i.e. aggressiveness, and extroversion that seem out of character), bizarre behavior, agitation, hallucinations, and depersonalization. Amnesia and other neuropsychiatric symptoms occur unpredictably, and in primarily depressed patients worsening of depression with suicidal thinking with the use of sedative/hypnotics.
Withdrawal: Withdrawal symptoms occur when stopped suddenly after daily use for a long time. In some cases, these symptoms can occur, even if used for only a week or two. In severe cases, abdominal and muscle cramps, vomiting, sweating, shakiness, and rarely, seizures occur. Rebound insomnia may occur when the medication is discontinued.
Drug Half-Life: 1 hour.

Stadol (brand) ~ Butorphanol (generic)

Common Usage: Narcotic analgesic—treatment of pain.

Action: Exact mechanism is unknown, but believed to attach to opiate receptors in the CNS.

Common Dosage: 1–4 mg I.M. (intramuscularly) with duration of 3–4 hours; 0.5–2 mg I.V. (intravenously) with duration of 2–4 hours; 1 mg nasally (1 spray in one nostril) with duration of 4 hours

Major Side Effects: Sedation, headache, severe dizziness, floating sensation, nervousness, lethargy, agitation, euphoria, hallucinations, flushing, palpitations, blood pressure changes, blurred vision, nausea, vomiting, dry mouth, rash, hives, excessive sweating, clammy skin, physical and mental dependence.

Interactions with Other Medications: Alcohol, CNS depressants potentiate CNS depression. Caution should be employed when drugs are combined.

Withdrawal: After administration as short as a month, withdrawal symptoms may occur with abrupt withdrawal. Symptoms may occur after the drug is withheld 4–12 hours. Symptoms include craving for the drug, insomnia, yawning, nausea, vomiting, sweating, tremors, diarrhea, mental depression, abdominal and muscle cramping/ aches, chills, and anxiety.

Drug Half-Life: 4.7–6.6 hours.

Strattera (brand) ~ Atomoxetine (generic)

Common Usage: Treatment of Attention Deficit/ Hyperactivity Disorder (ADHD).

Action: A selective norepinephrine reuptake inhibitor.

Common Dosage: *Dosing of children and adolescents up to 70 kg (< 150 pounds) body weight:* The total daily dose in children and adolescents should not exceed 1.4 mg/kg or 100 mg, whichever is less. No demonstrated benefits are seen with doses higher than 1.2 mg/kg/day.

216 / Break Your Prescribed Addiction

*Dosing of children and adolescents over 70 kg (over 150
pounds)* body weight and adults: 80 mg either administered as a single daily dose in morning, or as evenly divided doses in the morning and late afternoon/early evening.
The maximum recommended total daily dose in children
and adolescents over 70 kg and adults is 100 mg. No data
supports increased effectiveness at higher doses.

Contraindications: Not recommended in patients with
narrow angle glaucoma.

Major Side Effects: Can increase blood pressure and heart
rate, postural hypotension, increased urinary retention and
urinary hesitation, upper abdominal pain, vomiting, decrease in appetite, headache, somnolence, irritability, cough,
fatigue, insomnia, constipation, dry mouth, decreased libido,
ejaculatory problems, impotence, and dysmenorrhea.

Interactions with Other Medications: Strattera should
be administered with caution to patients being treated with
albuterol (or other beta$_2$ agonists) because the action of albuterol on the cardiovascular system can be potentiated.
Should not be taken with MAOI, or within two weeks after
discontinuing an MAOI. There have been reports of serious,
sometimes fatal reaction (including hyperthermia, rigidity,
myoclonus (a brief, sudden, singular, shock-like muscle contraction), autonomic instability with possible rapid fluctua-
tions of vital signs, and mental status changes that include
extreme agitation progressing to delirium and coma) when
taken in combination with a MAOI. Dosage adjustments may
be necessary when coadministered with paroxetine (Paxil),
fluoxetine (Prozac) and quinidine (an antiarrhythmic).

Precautions: Growth should be monitored during treatment; Strattera-treated patients lost an average of 0.4 kg,
while placebo patients gained an average of 1.5 kg; treated
patients grew an average of 0.9 cm, while placebo-treated
patients grew an average of 1.1 cm.

Drug Half-life: 5.2 hours in efficient metabolizers (EM) and 21.6 hours in poor metabolizers (PM).

Tegretol (brand) ~ Carbamazepine (generic)

Common Usage: Anticonvulsant used in the treatment of epilepsy, Trigeminal Neuralgia, and acute mania, and prophylaxis in bipolar disorder.
Action: Unknown, but is considered a tricyclic compound.
Common Dosage: 800–1200 mg daily.
Major Side Effects: leukopenia (low white blood cell count), elevated gamma-GT liver enzymes, skin sensitivity reactions and rashes, vertigo, somnolence, ataxia, fatigue, disturbances of cardiac conduction, bradycardia, arrhythmias, nausea, vomiting, edema.
Contraindications: Should not be administered to patients with a history of cardiac, hepatic disease, or renal damage, acute intermittent porphyria, or serious blood disorders. Should not be taken with or immediately following treatment with MAO inhibitor.
Precautions: Although reported infrequently, serious adverse effects have been observed during the use of carbamazepine. Agranulocytosis and aplastic anemia have occurred in a few instances resulting in death. Use this drug carefully. Close clinical and frequent laboratory supervision should be maintained throughout treatment in order to detect as early as possible signs and symptoms of a possible blood dyscrasia.
Drug Half-life: 16–24 hours.

Thorazine (brand)~ Chlorpromazine (generic)

Common Usage: Major tranquilizer/ antipsychotic and antiemetic.
Action: Thought to block the action of dopamine.
Common Dosage: 25–150 mg daily, in divided doses.

Major Side Effects: Dry mouth, blurred vision, constipation, impaired temperature regulation, orthostatic hypotension, and altered libido

Drug Interactions: Chlorpromazine may lower seizure threshold. Should not be taken with alcohol; use caution with amphetamines, second generation antihistamines, CNS depressants, anticholinergics, tricyclic antidepressants, levadopa, lithium.

Precautions: Neuroleptic malignant syndrome (NMS) has been reported with the use of chlorpromazine.

Withdrawal: Gastritis, nausea and vomiting, dizziness, and tremulousness, have been reported following abrupt cessation of high dose therapy. Reports suggest that these symptoms can be reduced if concomitant antiparkinsonian agents are continued for several weeks.

Drug Half-Life: 30 hours.

Tofanil (brand) ~ Imipramine (generic)

Common Usage: Tricyclic antidepressant, enuresis (bed wetting).

Action: Unknown, but believed to block reuptake of norepinephrine at nerve endings.

Common Dosage: 50–150 mg daily.

Major Side Effects: Dry mouth, drowsiness (especially when changing positions from sitting to rising or standing), dizziness, blurred vision, constipation, difficulty in urinating or urinary retention, weight gain, rapid pulse, hypertension. Extreme caution should be utilized in males with Benign Prostatic Hypertrophy (BPH), seizure disorders, thyroid problems, and narrow angle glaucoma.

Interactions with Other Medications: Do not take with alcohol or MAOs such as Nardil or Parnate. Combining imipramine with an MAO is dangerous and possibly fatal. Extreme caution should be used if imipramine is combined with antihypertensives (blood pressure medications) such as Catapres (clonidine), Ismelin (guanethidine), Tagamet (cimetidine), SSRIs (Prozac, Zoloft, Paxil, or Luvox), anticoagulants (Coumadin), Tegetrol (carbamazepine), Fastin (phentermine), Pondimin (fenfluramine), or decongestant/antihistamines.

Withdrawal: Abrupt withdrawal can cause nausea, headaches, weakness, and a sense of malaise.

Drug Half Life: 15–34 Hours; average 25 hours.

Topamax (brand) ~ Topiramate (generic)

Common Usage: Anticonvulsant

Action: Uncertain but believed to function as a sodium channel blocker, potentiate the action of GABA.

Common Dosage: Adults: 400 mg daily, in divided doses.

Major Side Effects: Somnolence, dizziness, ataxia, speech disorders, psychomotor slowing, nervousness, paresthesia, visual disorders/eye pain, memory difficulty, diplopia, fatigue, confusion, weight losss, language or mood problems. GI upset, anorexia, anxiety, kidney stones.

Drug Interactions: Phenytoin (Dilantin), carbamazepine (Tegretol), valproic (Depakote) acid reduce topiramate serum levels. Topiramate decreases serum levels of valproic acid. May increase phenytoin levels. May antagonize digoxin, oral contraceptives. CNS depression potentiated with alcohol, and other CNS depressants. Caution with other drugs that interfere with temperature regulation (e.g. anticholinergics, carbonic anhydrase inhibitors).

Precautions: Discontinue if acute myopia and secondary angle-closure glaucoma occurs. Hepatic or renal impairment, kidney stones, maintain adequate hydration and caloric intake, avoid ketogenic diets (low carbohydrate,

Atkins style diet), monitor closely for oligohidrosis (decreased sweating) and hyperthermia especially in children.
Withdrawal: Avoid abrupt cessation.
Drug Half-Life: 21 hours.

Tranxene (brand) ~ Clorazepate (generic)

Common Usage: Antianxiety—short-term anxiety and tension (less than 4 months; best 1-2 weeks; benzodiazepine.
Action: Depresses CNS in limbic system and promotes GABA transmission.
Common Dosage: 10–60 mg daily, divided.
Major Side Effects: Abuse potential, drowsiness, dizziness, light-headedness, fatigue, inability to concentrate, headache, memory impairment, unsteadiness, hangover, stupor, depression, nausea, slurred speech, constipation, salivary changes, incoordination, muscle movement, hiccups, ataxia (defective voluntary muscle coordination), menstrual irregularities, abnormal blood, liver and kidney tests, Paradoxical reaction (opposite reaction what drug is suppose to do)—excitement, rage, hallucinations, increased anxiety may occur in small number of people. Potential exists for abuse, both physical and psychological.
Interactions with Other Medications: Increased CNS depression is seen with alcohol and other CNS depressants such as narcotics and sedative-hypnotics. Cimetidine potentiates the sedative properties of clorazepate. Anti-Parkinson drugs such as levodopa may be less effect with clorazepate. Heavy smoking may reduce the effectiveness of clorazepate.
Withdrawal: Abrupt withdrawal symptoms may begin 2 to 6 days after last dosage, but can occur up to 10 days. Withdrawal symptoms include anxiety, irritability, insomnia, psychotic behavior, abdominal and muscle cramps,

hallucinations, convulsions, tremor, vomiting, sweating, insomnia, depression, restlessness, anxiety, unhappiness, general dissatisfaction. Sometimes delayed muscle spasms are seen days or weeks after all other withdrawal symptoms are gone.

Drug Half-Life: 30–200 hours.

Valium (brand) ~ Diazepam (generic)

Common Usage: Antianxiety—treatment of anxiety, tension; muscle relaxant, anticonvulsant, acute alcohol withdrawal syndrome, antipanic.

Action: Depresses the CNS in limbic system in brain. Valium is believed to increase the inhibitory neurotransmitter, GABA.

Common Dosage: 2–10 mg daily in divided dosages.

Major Side Effects: Dizziness, drowsiness, light-headedness, confusion, unsteadiness, headache, hangover, disorientation, insomnia, increased appetite, constipation, diarrhea, weight gain/loss, dry mouth, bitter/metallic taste, rash, itchy skin, increased or decreased libido, difficulty in urination, urinary retention, hyper/hypotension, pulse >100 or < 60, palpitations, abnormal blood tests, blurred vision, joint pains, muscle aches, shortness of breath.

Interactions with Other Medications: Alcohol, antihistamines, barbiturates, and phenothiazines potentiate CNS depressants leading to drowsiness, lethargy, stupor, respiratory collapse, coma, or death. Tricyclic antidepressants may add to sedative effects. Increased effects of benzodiazepines are seen with cimetidine, digoxin, phenytoin, probenecid, propoxyphene, propranolol, ketoconazole, fluoxetine, isoniazid, valproic acid, and erythromycin. Rantidine decreases absorption of benzodiazepines. Theophylline decreases sedative effects of benzodiazepines.

Withdrawal: Abrupt withdrawal after long-term use may produce anxiety, irritability, insomnia, psychotic behavior, convulsions, depression, hallucinations, sweating, vomiting, depression, restlessness, insomnia and severe abdominal and muscle cramps. Even after 4 to 6 weeks usage, withdrawal symptoms may be seen. But the withdrawal symptoms may not develop until 5 to 12 days after stopping diazepam, and may continue for days to weeks due to diazepam's long half-live. A tapered withdrawal over two weeks to a month is the best method to discontinue the drug.
Drug Half-Life: 20–70 hours.

Viagra (brand) ~ Sildenafil Citrate (generic)

Common Usage: Treatment of erectile dysfunction.
Action: Enhances the normal physiological action of nitric oxide.
Common Dosage: 25–100 mg.
Major Side Effects: headaches, facial flushing, upset stomach, bluish vision, decrease in supine blood pressure and sensitivity to light.
Drug Interactions: Viagra was shown to potentiate the hypotensive effects of nitrates and its administration in patients who use nitric oxide donors or nitrates in any form is therefore contraindicated. Use caution if taking alpha-blockers.
Precautions: Serious cardiovascular, cerebrovascular, and vascular events, including myocardial infarction, sudden cardiac death, ventricular arrhythmia, cerebrovascular hemorrhage (brain hemorrhage), transient ischemic attack (TIA), hypertension, subarachnoid and intracerebral hemorrhages (bleeds into the brain), and pulmonary (lung) hemorrhage have been reported post-marketing in temporal association with the use of Viagra. If an erection lasts

longer than four hours, seek immediate medical attention.
Drug Half-Life: 4 hours.

Others drugs for the treatment of erectile dysfunction include:

Cialis (brand) ~ Tadalafil (generic)

Levetra (brand) ~ Vardenafil (generic)

Muse (Brand) ~ Alprostadil (generic)

*Note-Researchers from Queen's University in Belfast have found evidence that the use of Viagra may impair fertility in men. If you are hoping to start a family, researchers advise that you do not take Viagra.

Vicodin (brand) ~ Hydrocodone (generic)

Common Usage: Narcotic analgesic—pain relief for moderate to moderately severe pain.

Action: Narcotic analgesics attach to opiate receptors in the CNS (spinal cord, brain, and brain stem) so analgesia results.

Common Dosage: 1 tablet every 4-6 hours.

Major Side Effects: Physical and psychological dependence, respiratory depression, lightheadedness, dizziness, headache, sedation, euphoria, mental clouding, fainting, restlessness, tremors, delirium, insomnia, nausea, vomiting, constipation, increased pressure in biliary tract, dry mouth, loss of appetite, flushing, changes in blood pressure and heart rate, skin rashes, sweating, urinary retention, reduced libido, changes in body temperature.

Interactions with Other Medications: Mixture of vicodin with alcohol, antihistamines, CNS depressants, methotrimeprazine, antianxiety, phenothiazines, sedative hypnotics, and skeletal muscle relaxants potentiate or add CNS depressant effects—drowsiness, lethargy, stupor, respiratory collapse, coma, or death. Addition of cimetidine may increase

CNS toxicity—disorientation, confusion, respiratory depression, apnea, and seizures. Tricyclic antidepressants increase narcotic induced respiratory depression.

Withdrawal: After the drug is withheld for 4 to 12 hours, withdrawal symptoms may arise. Symptoms include intense craving for the drug, insomnia, sneezing, yawning, nausea, vomiting, diarrhea, tremors, sweating, mental depression, abdominal pain, muscular aches and pains, chills, and anxiety.

Drug Half-Life: 3.8 hours.

Wellbutrin (brand) ~ Bupropion (generic)

Common Usage: Atypical depression, antidepressant. In addition, buproprion has been used to assist with nicotine withdrawal.

Action: Exact mechanism unknown, but weak reuptake of serotonin and norepinephrine, and to a lesser degree, dopamine.

Common Dosage: 100 mg, twice or three times daily.

Major Side Effects: Seizures, dizziness, rapid heart rate, rash, loss of appetite, constipation, nausea/vomiting, constipation, weight gain/loss, dry mouth, excessive sweating, headache/migraine, insomnia, sedation, confusion, tremor, agitation, restlessness, nervousness, rapid heartbeat, menstrual disturbance, fatigue, upper respiratory complaints.

Interactions with Other Medications: Avoid alcohol with buproprion. Never mix with other antidepressants, especially MAOIs. An increase in severity of side effects as well as reduction of dosage may be required if taking Levodopa, Dopar, Sinemet. Antihistamines like Hismanal and Seldane should not be combined with buproprion.

Withdrawal: Slow withdrawal over at least a 2-week period.

Drug Half Life: 3.9–24 hours.

Xanax (brand) ~ Alprazolam (generic)

Common Usage: Antianxiety with or without depression, panic disorder, benzodiazepine.

Action: Exact mechanism unknown, but depresses CNS in limbic system, and potentiates GABA transmission in the limbic system, hypothalamus and thalamus.

Common Dosage: 0.25–0.5 mg, three times daily.

Major Side Effects: Abuse potential, drowsiness, lightheadedness, depression, headache, dry mouth, constipation, diarrhea, nausea/vomiting, confusion, palpitation, heart rate > 100, increased salivation, hypotension (low blood pressure), blurred vision, muscular rigidity, tremors, nasal congestion, weight gain/loss, and blood test abnormalities.

Interactions with Other Medications: Additive CNS depressant effects are seen when combined with other psychotropic medications, anticonvulsants, antihistamines, alcohol and other drugs that depress the CNS. Increased levels of imipramine (Tofranil) and desipramine (Norpramin) are seen after adding alprazolam. Cimetidine delays the excretion of alprazolam and other benzodiazepines; the effects of alprazolam may be stronger.

Withdrawal: Abrupt withdrawal after an extended period of time may produce convulsions, tremor, abdominal and muscle cramps, vomiting, sweating, insomnia, depression, restlessness, anxiety, unhappiness, general dissatisfaction. Symptoms reported by patients after discontinuation of alprazolam include insomnia, lightheadedness, anxiety, fatigue, tiredness, abnormal involuntary movement, headache, nausea/vomiting, diarrhea, decreased salivation, weight loss, decreased appetite, sweating, rapid pulse > 100, blurred vision, muscular twitching.

Drug Half-Life: 6.3–26.9 hours.

Zoloft (brand) ~ Sertraline (generic)

Common Usage: SSRI, antidepressant, treatment of major depression.

Common Dosage: 25–200 mg per day.

Major Side Effects: Dry mouth, increased sweating, headache, dizziness, tremor, nausea, diarrhea, constipation, upset stomach, vomiting, flatulence, appetite loss, fatigue, insomnia, agitation, sleeplessness, sexual dysfunction (more incidence in males than females), anxiety, abnormal vision, and hot flashes.

Interactions With Other Medications: Do not take with alcohol. Over-the-counter drugs such as decongestants, antihistamines, or cold remedies may cause more side effects. Products containing tryptophan or 5HTP are not recommended, and may cause severe headaches, nausea, sweating and dizziness. Cimetidine (Tagamet) may increase the amount of Zoloft in the system, causing an increase in certain side effects. Increased bleeding times may be seen in patients taking warfarin (Coumadin). There may be a possibility of an interaction with sumitriptan (Imitrex), however, available studies have not been able to produce consistent results.

Withdrawal: Simply discontinue administration gradually over at least 2 weeks. After discontinuing any antidepressant depression symptoms may return. Seek professional help if depression returns. Withdrawal symptoms can begin 2 to 4 (and up to 7 days) after abrupt withdrawal. Abrupt withdrawal may include: nervousness, dizziness, insomnia, somnolence, nausea, flu-like syndrome without fever, loss of appetite, nausea, vomiting, upset stomach, sweating, anxiety, agitation, irritability, rapid heart beat, tension headache, neckache, chills, malaise, runny nose, somnolence, excessive dreaming, nightmares, vertigo

(dizziness) often with vomiting, visual distortions, and migraine-like headache.
Drug Half-Life: 26 hours.

Zomig (brand) ~ Zolmitriptan (generic)

Common Usage: Relieve migraines, but does not prevent or reduce number of attacks.
Action: Exact mechanism is unknown, but binds to 5-HT receptors in the brain.
Common Dosage: 1.25-2.5 mg with onset of headache, and second dose after 2 hours of administration the first dose if headache returns. Do not take more than a total of 10 mg in any 24 hour period. If first dosage does not reduce or relieve pain, do not take a second dosage.
Major Side Effects: Tightness in the chest or throat, shortness of breath, wheezing, heart throbbing, swelling of eyelids, face or lips, skin rash, skin lumps, hives, tingling, heat, heaviness or pressure after treatment, drowsiness, dizziness, fatigue or feeling sick.
Interactions with Other Medications: None known.
Withdrawal: Usually none as the medication should only be used on an as needed basis. No tolerance or withdrawal should occur with occasional usage.
Drug Half-Life: 2–5 hours.

Zyban: See Wellbutrin.

Zyprexa (brand) ~ Olanzapine (generic)

Common Usage: Antipsychotic; treatment of schizophrenia and psychoses.
Action: Exact mechanism is unknown, but believed to increase dopamine, serotonin, GABA, and histamine levels.
Common Dosage: 5–10 mg per day.

Major Side Effects: Sedation, dizziness, weight gain, personality disorder, rapid heartbeats, decrease in blood pressure, runny nose, nervousness, agitation, sleepiness, tremor, rigid muscles, weakness, constipation, drowsiness.

Interactions with Other Medications: Avoid alcohol. When combined with alcohol or diazepam (Valium), severe dizziness and hypotension (decreased blood pressure) with fainting. If combined with SSRIs (Luvox, Zoloft, Paxil, Prozac, Serzone, or Effexor) as well as other antipsychotics, severity of side effects may be increased. Antihypertensive medications in combination with olanzapine may produce increased dizziness due to drop in blood pressure. Possible interactions may occur (unproven at this time) with phentermine (Fastin), fenfluramine (Pondimin), dexfenfluramine (Redux), and sumatriptan (Imitrex). Symptoms may include sudden agitation and restlessness. Faster excretion of olanzapine may occur with carbamazepine (Tegretol), omeprazole (Prilosec), and rifampin (Rafadin).

Withdrawal: Abrupt withdraw can cause insomnia, aggravated feeling of depression and unrest without cause, convulsions, tremor, abdominal and muscle cramping, vomiting, and sweating.

Precautions: Hyperglycemia and/or diabetes with ketoacidosis, coma, and death associated with use of clozapine.

Drug Half-Life: 21–54 hours.

Checklist Of Addictive And Behavior Characteristics

- [ ] 1. Alcohol and nicotine dependence.
- [ ] 2. Attends clinic without family support.
- [ ] 3. Visits multiple physicians.
- [ ] 4. Lives on welfare and disability.
- [ ] 5. Avoids eye contact with health care
- [ ] practitioner.
- [ ] 6. Refuses psychotherapy.
- [ ] 7. Avoids group sessions.
- [ ] 8. Needs prescription refills ahead of schedule.
- [ ] 9. Complains of falling and pain.
- [ ] 10. Does not have primary care physician.
- [ ] 11. Positive urine test for marijuana, cocaine, methamphetamines, or alcohol.
- [ ] 12. Reports medication or prescription lost or stolen.
- [ ] 13. Inconsistent or false medical records.
- [ ] 14. Refuses lab or diagnostic tests.
- [ ] 15. Spends excessive time in clinic.
- [ ] 16. Requests dosage increase of medications.
- [ ] 17. Visits ER frequently.
- [ ] 18. Requests short acting opioids.
- [ ] 19. No employment history.
- [ ] 20. Does not keep appointments and reschedules.
- [ ] 21. Not interested in pain or stress management group.

List Of Practitioners
That Practice Nutritional Medicine

Annemarie Welch, M.D.
2301 W. Hwy 89A, Suite 104
Sedona, AZ 86336
(928) 282-0609

The Amen Clinic
350 Chadbourne Rd.
Fairfield, CA 84585
(707) 429–7181

Daniel Amen, M.D.
The Amen Clinic
4001 Westerly Place Suite 108
Newport Beach, CA 92660
(949) 266-3700

Alice Feldman, M.D.
299 El Camino Real
Millbrae, CA 94030
(650) 692–1816

Paul Lynn, M.D.
345 W. Portal Suite 2
San Francisco, CA 94127
(415) 566-1000

Phyllis Bronson, Ph.D.
100 E. Main Street
Aspen, CO 81611
(573) 778–0500

Marcy Foley, N.D.
Kornax Enterprises
11982 Twilight St.
Longmont, CO 80503
(303) 823–5813

Jim Denney, N.D.
3424 Vineville Ave.
Macon, GA 31204
(478) 476–9954

Linda Griffith, R.N.
Bio Scan of Boise
4274 Wisteria Way
Boise, ID 83713
(208) 377-3762

W.R. Elghammer, M.D.
723 N. Logan Ave. #1
Danville, IL 61832
(217) 446–3259

Laurie Allen, D.C.
Allen Chiropractic
2725 N. Westwood Blvd. #5B
Poplar Bluff, MO 63901
(970) 920–2523

Natalie Sadler, M.D.
P.O. Box 2070
Chapel Hill, NC 27515
(919) 929-7527

Joan Nielsen, M.D.
218 Rosebrook Dr.
Cary, NC 27513
(919) 467–5770

Jacqueline Krohn, M.D.
3917 West Rd. #136
Los Alamos, NM 87544
(505) 662–9620

Sherry A. Rogers, M.D.
2800 W. Genesee St.
Syracuse, NY 13219
(315) 488–2856

The Amen Clinic
3315 S. 23rd St.
Tacoma, WA 98405
(253) 779–4673

Andy Vorster, M.D.
National Health Associates
2205 Portsmouth St.
Houston, TX 77098
(713) 528–8600

Todd Goodale, D.C.
1833 El Dorado Blvd.
Houston, TX 77062
(281) 480–7784

Dennis Remington, M.D.
1675 N. Freedom Blvd.
Provo, UT 84604
(801) 373-8500

Julie Davis, N.C.
Utah Valley Health Clinic
3311 N. University Ave
Suite 100
Provo, UT 84604
(801) 374-5667

Martin Feldman, M.D.
132 E 76th St. Office 1A
New York, NY 10021
(212) 744-4413

The Amen Clinic
1875 Campus Commons Dr.
Ste. 101
Reston, VA 20191
(703) 860–5600

Kary Chiropractic Center
660 Jadwin Ave. Suite A
Richland, WA 99352
(509) 943–5314

Top 200 Drugs For 2003
by Number of Prescriptions Dispensed
Source: *NDC Health*

1. Hydrodone w/APAP
2. Lipitor (Atorvastatin)
3. Synthroid (Levothyroxine)
4. Tenoretic (Atenolo)
5. Zithromax (Azithromycin)
6. Amoxicillin (generic)
7. Lasix (Furosemide)
8. Hyzaar (Hydrochlorothiazide)
9. Norvasc (Amlodipine)
10. Lisinopril (generic)
11. Xanax (Alprazolam)
12. Zoloft (Sertraline)
13. Albuterol Aerosol (Albuterol)
14. Toprol-XL (Metoprolol)
15. Zocor (Simvastatin)
16. Premarin (Conjugated Estrogens)
17. Prevacid (Lansoprazole)
18. Zyrtec (Cetirizine)
19. Ibuprofen (generic)
20. Levoxyl (Levothyroxine)
21. Propoxyphene N /APAP (generic)
22. Triamterene/HCTZ (generic)
23. Celebrex (Celecoxib)
24. Ambien (Zolpidem)
25. Allegra (Fexofenadine)
26. Cephalexin (generic)
27. Nexium (Esomeprazole)
28. Fosamax (Alendronate)
29. Vioxx (Rofecoxib)
30. Singulair (Montelukast)
31. Ortho Tri-Cyclen (Norgestimate /Ethinyl Estradiol)
32. Prednisone (generic)
33. Meroprolol Tartrate (generic)
34. Prozac (Fluoxetine)
35. Effexor XR (Venlafaxine)
36. Neurontin (Gabapentin)
37. Ativan (Lorazepam)
38. Klonopin (Clonazepam)
39. Celexa (Citalopram)
40. Viagra (Sildenafil Citrate)
41. Wellbutrin SR (Bupropion HCl)
42. Paxil (Paroxetine)
43. Pravachol (Pravastatin)
44. Plavix (Clopidogrel)
45. Trimox (Amoxicillin)
46. Potassium Chloride (generic)
47. Protonix (Pantoprazole)
48. Advair Diskus (Salmeterol/Fluticasone)
49. Flonase (Fluticasone)
50. Glucophage (Metformin)
51. Amoxicillin/Clavulante (generic)
52. Elavil (Amitriptyline)
53. Zantac (Ranitidine)
54. Acetaminiphen/Codeine (generic)
55. Lexapro (Escitalopram)
56. Accupril (Quinapril)
57. Levaquin (Levofloxacin)
58. Altace (Ramipril)
59. Diovan (Valsartan)
60. Lotrel (Amlodipine/Benazepril)
61. Warfarin (generic)
62. Prilosec (Omeprazole)
63. Flexeril (Cyclobenzaprine)
64. Glucotrol XL (Glipizide)
65. Diflucan (Fluconazole)
66. Verapamil (generic)
67. Bextra (Valdecoxib)
68. Penicillin VK (generic)
69. Cozarr (Losartan)
70. Actos (Pioglitazone)
71. Trazodone (generic)
72. Glyburide (generic)
73. Naproxen (generic)
74. Diovan HCT (Valsartan/HCTZ)
75. Coumadin (Warfarin)
76. Ortho Evra (Norelgestromin/Ethinyl Estradiol)
77. Avandia (Rosiglitazone maleate)
78. Paxil (Paroxetine)
79. Risperdal (Risperidone)
80. Flomax (Tamsulosin)
81. Aciphex (Rabeprazole)
82. Digitek (Digoxin)
83. Cipro (Ciprofloxacin)
84. Nasonex (Mometasone)
85. Oxycodone /APAP (generic)
86. Glucophage XR (Metformin)
87. Lotensin (Benazepril)
88. Evista (Raloxifene)
89. Zyprexa (Olanzapine)
90. Diltiazem HCI (generic)
91. Allegra-D (Fexofenadine /Pseudoephedrine)
92. Clonidine (generic)
93. Lanoxin (Digoxin)
94. Hyzaar (Losartan / HCTZ)
95. Amoxil (Amoxicillin)
96. Actonel (Risedronate)

97. Oxycontin (Oxycodone)
98. Cotrim (Trimeth/Sulfameth)
99. Xalatan (Latanoprost)
100. Tricor (Fenofibrate)
101. Amaryl (Glimepiride)
102. Concerta (Methlphenidate XR)
103. Flovent (Fluticasone Propionate)
104. Glucovance (Glyburide/Metformin)
105. Combivent (Ipratropium/Albuterol)
106. Adderall XR (Amphetamine Mixed Salts)
107. Prilosec (Omeprazole)
108. Seroquel (Quetiapine)
109. Yasmin 28 (Drospirenone/Ethinyl Estradiol)
110. Valtrex (Valacyclovir)
111. Depakote (Divalproex)
112. Prempro (Conj. Estrogens/ Medroxyprogesterone)
113. Carisoprodol (Carisoprodol)
114. Isosorbide Mononitrate (generic)
115. Levothroid (Levothyroxine)
116. Avapro (Irbesartan)
117. Diazepam (generic)
118. Detrol LA (Tolterodine)
119. Humulin N (Human Insulin NPH)
120. Lantus (Insulin Glargine)
121. Coreg (Carvedilol)
122. Enalapril (generic)
123. Ultracet (Tramadol/Acetaminophen)
124. Promethazine (generic)
125. Endocet (Oxycodone/APAP)
126. Gemfibrozil (generic)
127. Topamax (Topiramate)
128. Skelaxin (Metaxalone)
129. Biaxin XL (Clarithromycin)
130. Cartia XT (Diltiazem)
131. Monopril (Fosinopril)
132. Zetia (Ezetimibe)
133. Folic Acid (generic)
134. Rhinocort Aqua (Budesonide)
135. Omnicef (Cefdinir)
136. Meclizine (generic)
137. Nasacort AQ (Triamcinolone Acetonide)
138. Augmentin ES600 (Amoxicillin /Clavulante)
139. Macrobid (Nitrofurantoin)
140. Temazepam (generic)
141. Doxycycline Hyclate (Doxycycline)
142. Imitrex (Sumatriptan)
143. Necon (Ethinyl Estradio/Norethindrone)
144. Klor-Con (Potassium Chloride)
145. Klor-Con M20 (Potassium Chloride)
146. Allopurinol (generic)
147. Dilantin (Phenytoin)
148. SMZ-TMP (Trimeth/Sulfameth)
149. Microgestin Fe (Norethindrone/Ethinyl Estradiol)
150. Humalog (Insulin Lispro)
151. Cefzil (Cefprozil)
152. Duragesic (Fentanyl)
153. Bactroban (Mupirocin)
154. Patanol (Olopatadine)
155. Humulin 70/30 (Human Insulin 70/30)
156. Aricept (Donepezil)
157. Miralax (PEG 3350)
158. Aviane (Levonorgestrel/Ethinyl Estradiol)
159. Zyrtec-D (Cetirizine/Pseudoephedrine)
160. Ditropan XL (Oxybutynin)
161. Biaxin (Clarithromycin)
162. Ciprofloxacin (generic)
163. Niaspan (Niacin)
164. Strattera (Atomoxetine)
165. Inderal LA (Propranolol)
166. Elidel (Pimecrolimus)
167. Pulmicort (Budesonide)
168. Trivora-28 (Levonorgestrel /Ethinyl Estradiol)
169. Albuterol (generic)
170. Nifedipine ER (generic)
171. Methylprednisolone (generic)
172. Tussionex (Hydrocodone/Chlorpheniramine)
173. Mobic (Meloxicam)
174. Timolol (generic)
175. Atacand (Candesartan)
176. Phenytoin (generic)
177. Alphagan P (Brimonidine)
178. Avelox (Moxifloxacin)
179. Clorimazole / Betamethasone (generic)
180. Triamcinolone (generic)
181. Lescol XL (Fluvastatin)
182. Miacalcin (Calcitonin)
183. Ortho-Novum (Norethindrone/Ethinyl Estradiol)
184. Plendil (Felodipine)
185. Promethazine / Codeine (generic)
186. Nitroquick (Nitroglycerin)
187. Spironolactone (generic)
188. Terazosin (generic)
189. Proscar (Finasteride)
190. Avalide (Irbesartan /HCTZ)
191. Kariva (Desogestrel / Ethinyl Estradiol)
192. Low-Ogestrel (Norgestrel/Ethinyl Estradiol)
193. Tobradex (Tobramycin/ examethasone)
194. Remeron (Mirtazapine)
195. Roxicet (Oxycodone/Acetaminophen)
196. Percocet (Oxycodone/Acetaminophen)
197. Atrovent (Ipratropium)
198. Propranolol (generic)
199. Nifediac CC (Nifedipine)
200. Apri (Disogestrel / Ethinyl Estradiol)

Vitamins And Nutrients That Aid Recovery From Drugs/Substance Abuse

Nutrient	Usage	Therapeutic Dosage
Vitamin E	Detoxification, Antioxidant.	Start with 400 I.U., then increase to 800 I.U. after 2 weeks, and continue daily.
Ester C	Detoxification.	2,000 to 5,000 mg daily
B Complex	Important for the nervous system. Important cofactor in many body enzyme reactions.	1 daily
B6	Activation of amino acids and nutrients.	1 (150 mg) timed-release cap
Mag Link	Activation of amino acids, proper mental function.	2 caps, 2 to 3 times daily
Multiple Vitamin (T-L Vite)	Replenishes deletion. Replenishes body.	1 with main meal
Anxiety Control *OR*	Anti-anxiety formula.	1 or 2, 3 times throughout the day
GABA 750	Antistress. Anxiety.	Dissolve in 6–8 oz. of water, 2 to 3 times daily. Must be pure GABA. *Do not megadose.*
Tyrosine	Depression.	850 mg, 2 to 3 times daily, spread out.
L–T	Creates alpha waves (like deep relaxation).	200 mg, twice daily.
Brain Link	Neurotransmitter/nutrient support, replenishes exhausted amino acids and neurotransmitters.	2 scoops, 3 times daily.
Super B.N.C.	Provides a balance of amino acids to restore brain and body chemistry.	2 capsules, 3 times daily
Glutamine	Anticraving, antistress. Elevates serotonin, GABA, dopamine.	1,000 mg powder, 3 times daily, dissolved in water.
Mood Sync	Anti-stress, anti-anxiety.	1–2 caps, 2 to 3 times daily
Green Tea Extract	Antioxidant, super immune enhancer.	1 (500 mg); 2, if needed.
DHA-EPA (ProDHA)	Mood stabilizer.	2 caps, 2 times daily.

Amino Acids And Nutrients For Clinical Conditions And Diseases

The following list is only a guideline for specific conditions. Each individual's needs are different. Some nutrients will help you more than others. Therefore, you must find the nutrients that best suit your situation.

Condition	Suggested Therapy	Avoid
Aging	Methionine, 5-HTP, Glutamine, Ester C, Super BNC, Melatonin, Decaf Green Tea Ext	
Aggressiveness	5-HTP, GABA , Glycine, Glutamine, Taurine, Tyrosine, B6, BNC + GABA, Liquid Serotonin, Mag Chlor 85/Mag Link	Phenylalanine
Alzheimer's	BNC + GABA, Glutamine, Ginkgo B6 (Timed Release), Decaf Green Tea Ext. Vinpocetine, Huperzine A, ProDHA,	
Arthritis	BNC + GABA,Boswella, Glucosamine, Malic Acid +, DLPA, Ester C, Magnesium, Niacinamide, Histidine, Cysteine,	
Autism	5-HTP, Glutamine, B6, Taurine, Liquid Serotonin, Magnesium, Brain Link	
Body Building	BCAA, Alanine, Carnitine	
Cancer	Cysteine, Taurine, Glutamine, Super BNC, Ester C, Decaf Green Tea Extract BCAA, Melatonin, Beta Glucan	With Melanoma Phenylalanine, Tyrosine
Cholesterol	Carnitine, Methionine, Arginine, Glycine, Taurine, Fortified Flax, Chromium Pic, ProDHA, Policosanol	
Chronic Illness	BCAA, Super BNC, Decaf Green Tea Ext., Cystine, 5-HTP, Ester C, Pycnogenol	
Chronic Pain	5-HTP, DLPA , GABA, Glutamine, MSM, Super BNC, Boswella, Ester C, ProDHA Mag Link or Mag Chlor 85, Pain Control	
Cirrhosis / G.I. Healing	Glutamine, Carnitine, BCAA, Milk Thistle, CoEnzyme Q10, Glutamine, Beta Glucan	
Depression	5-HTP, Phenylalanine or Tyrosine, Taurine Methionine, GABA, Carnitine, Threonine, Mood Sync, Mag Link or Mag Chlor 85, ProDHA	
Diabetes	5-HTP, Carnitine, Taurine, Chromium Pic, Vitamin E, Mag Link, Vanadium, Decaf Green Tea Extract, Alpha Lipoic Acid, Ester C,	
Drug Addiction	GABA , Methionine, Tyrosine, ProDHA, Glutamine, DLPA, B Complex, 5-HTP, B6 (Timed Release), Super BNC	Alcohol
Energy	Carnitine, Tyrosine, CoEnzyme Q10	Melatonin

Epilepsy	L–T, Taurine, GABA, B6, Mag Chlor	
Gallbladder	Methionine, Taurine, Glycine, BCAA	
Gout	Glycine, MSM	
Heart Failure	Taurine, Tyrosine, Carnitine, BCAA, CoEnzyme Q10, Mag Link or Mag Chlor	
Herpes	Lysine, Ester C, Zinc, Beta Glucan	
Hyperactivity	GABA, Glycine, Glutamine, Taurine, 5-HTP, Liq.Serotonin, Super BNC or Brain Link	
Hypertension	5-HTP, GABA, Taurine, Mag Link, Mag Link or Mag Chlor, CoEnzyme Q10	
Hypoglycemia	Alanine, GABA, Chromium Picolinate, Mag Link or Mag Chlor	
Insomnia	5-HTP, Melatonin or Sleep Link, Mag Chlor Liquid Serotonin, GABA,	Phenylalanine
Kidney Failure	BNC + GABA, Carnitine,	
Leg Ulcers	Topical Cysteine, Glycine, Threonine, BCAA, Ester C, Zinc, Magnesium	
Liver Disease	BCAA, Carnitine, Glutamine, B6	
Manic	5-HTP, GABA, Glycine, Super BNC, GABA Glutamine, Lithium, Mag Chlor 85	Phenylalanine
Memory/ Concentration	Glutamine, GABA, Super BNC, Huperzine, Ginkgo, Vinpocetine, B6 (Timed Release)	
Mental Alertness	Tyrosine, Phenylalanine, Glutamine, Ginkgo	
Parkinson's	Phenylalanine, Tyrosine, 5-HTP, Methionine, Mag Link or Mag Chlor, Ester C, Super BNC	
Radiation	Cysteine, Glutamine, Taurine, Ester C, Beta Carotene, Decaf Green Tea Extract, Beta Glucan	
Schizophrenia	GABA, Isoleucine, 5-HTP, Methionine, B6, ProDHA, Niacin	Serine, Leucine Aspargine
Seizures /Tics	Taurine, GABA, Mag Link or Mag Chlor	
Stress	Tyrosine, GABA, Histidine, Super BNC, Glutamine, B6, Glycine, Ester C, Mag Link or Mag Chlor	
Surgery	BCAA, Super BNC, Glutamine, Ester C, Beta Carotene	
Tardive Dyskinesia	GABA, Taurine, BCAA, Glutamine, Mag Link or Mag Chlor	
Tobacco Addiction	Tyrosine, GABA , 5HTP, or Mood Sync, Glutamine, Methionine, B Complex, Sulfonil	
Weight Control	5-HTP, Phenylalanine, GABA, Tyrosine, HCA	

Amino acids are involved in many metabolic pathways in the body. They are extremely important as detoxifying and immune stimulating agents. Detoxifying amino acids include cysteine, glutamine, glycine, methionine, taurine and tyrosine. Immunostimulating amino acids include: alanine, aspartic acid, cysteine, glycine, lysine and threonine.

Drug-Nutrient Actions

Drug/ Condition	Parallel Nutrient	Opposite Nutrient
Anticonvulsants	Taurine, GABA, Glycine, 5-HTP Magnesium	Aspartic Acid
Antidepressants	Phenylalanine Tyrosine Methionine Taurine 5-HTP or Tryptophan	Glycine, Histidine
Heart Failure	Taurine CoEnzyme Q10 Carnitine Mag Link	Niacinamide 5-HTP
High Cholesterol / Triglycerides	Carnitine, Chromium Picolinate	
Steroids (anabolic)	BCAA, Carnitine	Glutamic Acid
Viral antagonists	Lysine, Zinc	Arginine

For Product Information Call 1-800-669-2256
or
visit http://www.painstresscenter.com

Bibliography

Abbott, F.V. and M.I. Fraser. "Use and abuse of over-the-counter analgesic agents." *Journal of Psychiatry Neuroscience.* January 1998, Vol. 23 No. 1, pp. 13–34.

Adams, Ruth and Frank Murray. *Megavitamin Therapy.* New York: Larchmont Books, 1980.

Adour, K., R. Hilsinger, and F. Byl. *American Otolaryngology Annual Meeting Review Notes.* Dallas, Texas. October 7–11, 1985.

"Advancing the Frontiers of Drug Abuse Research." *NIDA (National Institute of Drug Abuse, 1975–2004.* U.S. Dept. of Health and Human Services, National Institute of Health, pp. 5, 8.

Advisor Forum. "Benzodiazepine Withdrawal Time." *Clinical Advisor.* February 1998, p. 56.

Agren, H., et al. "Low brain uptake of L-5-hydroxytryptophan in major depression: A positron emission tomography study on patients and healthy volunteers." *Acta Psychiatry Scan.* Vol. 83, 1991, pp. 449–455.

Angell, Marcia and Arnold S. Relman. " *Prescription for Profit.*" *The Washington Post*, June 20, 2001, p. A27.

Angell, Marcia. "The Pharmaceutical Industry—To Whom Is It Accountable?" *The New England Journal of Medicine*, June 22, 2000, pp. 1902–1904.

Angst J. et al. "The treatment of depression with l-5-hydroxytryptophan versus imipramine: Results of two open and one double-blind study." *Arch Psychiatry Nervenkr.* Vol. 224, 1977, pp. 175–186.

Ashton, C. Heather. *Benzodiazepines How They Work & How to Withdraw.* Newcastle, England: University of Newcastle, School of Neurosciences, Division of Psychiatry, August 2002.

Asnis, G.M., S.R. Kohn, M. Henderson, N.L. Brown. "SSRIs versus non-SSRIs in post traumatic stress disorder: an update with recommendations." *Drugs.* Vol. 64, No. 4, pp. 383–404. Review.

Atal. C.K., Gupto O.P., Raghunathan, K., Dhar, K.l. "Pharmacognosy and Phytochemistry of Withania Somnifers", *Central Council for Research In Indian Medicine and Homeopathy*: New Delhi, 1975.

Barbeau, A. *Archives Neurology.* Vol. 30. (1982), pp. 52–58.

Basbaum, A.I. and H.L. Fields. "Endogenous pain control mechanisms: review and hypothesis." *Annuals of Neurology.* Vol. 4, 1978, pp. 451–462.

Beckmann, H., D. Athen, M. Oheanu, and R. Zimmer. "DL-phenylalanine Versus Imipramine: A Double Blind Controlled Study." *Archives Psychiatric Nervenkr.* Vol. 227 (1979).

Benowitz, Neal L. "Pharmacologic Aspects of Cigarette Smoking and Nicotine Addiction." *The New England Journal of Medicine.* Nov. 17, 1988.

Bergland, Richard. *The Fabric of the Mind.* New York: Viking Penguin, Inc., 1985, pp. 80-98.

Berman, J. R. "Progabide, A New GABA Mimetric Agent in Clinical Use." *Clinical Neuropharmacology,* 1985.

Blier, P. "Norepinephrine and selective norepinephrine reuptake inhibitors in depression and mood disorders: their pivotal role." *Journal of Psychiatry Neurosciences.* 2001, Vol. 26 (Supp): S1–2. Abstract.

Blum, Kenneth. *Handbook of Abusable Drugs.* New York: Gardner Press, Inc., 1984, pp. 5, 205.

Blum, Kenneth and Michael C. Trachtenberg. *Some Things You Should Know About Alcoholism.* Houston, Texas: MATRIX Technologies, Inc., 1988.

Bond, Michael. *Pain, Its Nature, Analysis, and Treatment.* New York: Churchill Livingstone, 1979), p. 102.

Booker, Jack E. "Pain It's All in Your Patient's Head (Or is It?)." *Nursing 82.* March, pp. 47-51.

Borison, et al. "Metabolism of the Antidepressant Amino Acid, L-phenylalanine." *Fellows of American Society of Experimental Biology Meeting Notes.* April 9-14, 1978.

Borum, P. R. *Annual Review Nutrition.* Vol. 3 (1983), pp. 233-259.

Borum, P. R. *Nutrition Review.* Vol. 39 (1981), pp. 285-390.

Braverman, Eric R. and Carl C. Pfeiffer. *The Healing Nutrients Within: Facts, Findings and the New Research on Amino Acids.* New Canaan, Connecticut: Keats Publishing Co., Inc., 1987, pp. 8, 12–13, 24, 29–58, 120–127, 306–314, 330–331.

Breggin, Peter R., M.D. *Brain Disabling Treatments in Psychiatry*, New York, NY: Springer Publishing Company Inc. 1997.

Breggin, Peter R. "Fluvoxamine as a cause of stimulation, mania and aggression with a critical analysis of FDA approval label." *International Journal of Risk and Safety in Medicine*. Vol. 14., 2001, pp. 71–86.

Breggin, Peter R. "Suidicality, violence and mania caused by selective serotonin reuptake inhibitors (SSRIs): A review and analysis." *International Journal of Risk and Safety in Medicine*. Vol. 16, 2003/2004, pp. 31–49.

Breggin, Peter R., M.D. *Toxic Psychiatry*. New York: St. Martin's Press, 1994.

Breggin, Peter R., M.D. *Talking Back to Prozac*. NewYork: St. Martin's Press, 1994.

Brenton, Myron and eds. *Emotional Health*. Emmaus, PA: Rodale Press, 1985, p. 129.

Bresler, David E. with Richard Trubo. *Free Yourself From Pain*. New York: Simon and Schuster, 1979, p. 298.

Chaitow, Leon. *Amino Acids in Therapy*. Rochester, Vermont: Thorsons Publishers, Inc., 1985.

Challem, Jack. *The Inflammation Syndrome*, Hoboken, New Jersey: John Wiley & Sons, Inc., 2003.

Cherchi, A. et al. *American Journal of Cardiology*. Vol. 33 (1979), pp. 300-306.

Chilnick, Lawrence D., ed., et. Al. *The Pill Book of Anxiety and Depression*. New York: Bantam Books, 1985.

Cooper, J. R., F.E. Bloom, and R.H. Roth, eds. *The Biochemical Basis of Neuropharmacology*, 7th ed. New York: Oxford University Press, 1996.

Cohen, Jay S, M.D. *Over Dose, The Case Against the Drug Companies*. New York, NY: Penguin Putnam, 2001.

Colombetti, G. and S. Monti. *European Physiology Congress Proceedings*. 1st Quarter, No. 2. 1971, pp. 45–53.

Colvin, Rod. *Prescription Drug Addiction*. Omaha, NE: Addicus Books, 2002.

Consumer Reports; January 1993.

Conquer JA, Tierney MC, Zecevic J, et al. "Fatty acid analysis of blood plasma of patients with Alzheimer's disease, other types of dementia, and cognitive impairment." *Lipids* Vol. 35. No. 1, 2000, pp. 305–12.

Dean, Carolyn, M.D., N.D., *The Miracle of Magnesium*. New York, NY: Ballantine Books, 2003.

Detke, M.J., Y. Lu, et al. "Fuloxetine, 60 mg once daily for major depressive disorder: a randomixed double blind placebo controlled trial." *Journal of Clinical Psychiatry*. Vol 63. 1998, pp. 308–315.

Devlin, T. M. *Textbook of Biochemistry*. New York: Wiley Press, 1982.

Diamond, Seymour and Jose Medina. "Headaches." *Clinical Symposia*. Vol. 33, No. 2 (1981).

Dietrich, Schneider-Helmert. "Interval Therapy with L-tryptophan in Severe Chronic Insomniacs," *International Pharmacopsychiatry*. Vol. 16 (1981), pp. 162-173.

Emergency Dept. (ED) mentions for selected drug categories, total ED drug episodes and mentions, and total ED visit: Estimates for the coterminous U.S. by year. Table 2.2.0. Emergency Departments from Drug Abuse Warning Network (DAWN) series D-24, Publications No. (SMA) 03-3780 Rockville, MD. 08/2003.

Emergency Dept. (ED) mentions for selected major substances of abuse by drug category: Estimates for the coterminous U.S. by year. Table 2.4.0. Emergency Departments from Drug Abuse Warning Network (DAWN) series D-24, Publications No. (SMA) 03-3780 Rockville, MD. 08/2003

Emergency Dept. (ED) mentions for psychotherapeutic agents by drug cateselected drug categories: Estimates for the coterminous U.S. by year. Table 2.6.0. Emergency Departments from Drug Abuse Warning Network (DAWN) series D-24, Publications No. (SMA) 03-3780 Rockville, MD. 08/2003.

Eisner, Robin. "Falling Off Prozac." *ABC News*, 2000.

Essman, W. B., ed. *Nutrients and Brain Function*. Switzerland: Karger, 1987, pp. 2-3, 164.

Farquharson, J. Infant cerebral cortex and dietary fatty acids. *European Journal of Clinical Nutrtion*. Vol. 48, S2, 1994.

Feldberg and Hetzel. *Food Technology*. Vol. 12 (1958).

Finnegan, John and Daphne Gray. *Recovery from Addiction*. Berkley, CA: Celestial Arts, 1975.

Fischer, E., H. Spatz, J. M. Saaverdra, H. Reggiani, A. H. Miro, and B. Heller. "Urinary Elimination of Phenylethylamine." *Biological Psychiatry*. Vol. 2, No. 2 (1972).

Fishbain, D. "Evidence-based data on pain relief with antidepressants." *Annuals Medicine*. Vol. 32, pp. 305–316.

Ford, Regina Daley, Ed. *MediQuik Cards*. Springhouse, PA: Springhouse Corporation, 1988.

Fox, Arnold and Barry Fox. *DLPA, To End Chronic Pain and Depression*. New York: Pocket Books, 1985, pp. 147–199.

Frawley, David, N.D. "Ashwagandha is the Great Tonic of Ayurveda." *Lets's Live*, December 1993, p. 80.

Fruton, Joseph and Sofia Simmonds. *General Biochemistry*. New York: Wiley, 1958, p. 792.

Gaby, Alan. *B-6, The Healing Nutrient*. New Canaan, Connecticut: Keats Publishing, Inc., 1984, pp. 58-62.

Gallagher, R.M. and S. Verma. "Managing pain and comorbid depression: a public health challenge. *Seminars of Clinical Neuropsychiatry*. Vol. 4, 1999, pp. 203–220.

Gant, Charles and Greg Lewis. *End Your Addiction Now*. New York, NY: Warner Books, 2002.

Garrett, R. C. and U. G. Waldmeyer. *The Pill Book of Anxiety and Depression*. New York: Bantam Books, 1985, p. 9.

Garrison, Robert Jr. *Lysine, Tryptophan, and Other Amino Acids*. (New Canaan, Connecticut: Keats Publishing, Co., Inc., 1982), pp. 2–9.

Garzya, G. and R. M. Amico. *International Journal Tissue Reactions*. Vol. 11 (1980), pp. 175–180.

Gelenberg, Alan J. et al. "Tyrosine for the Treatment of Depression." *American Journal of Psychiatry*. (May 1980), pp. 622-623.

Gerald, Michael C., *Pharmacology, An Introduction to Drugs*. (New York: Prentice-Hall, 1981), pp. 30–31.

Gerber, Harris, and Frizzel. "Treatment of Rheumatoid Arthritis with Histidine—A Double Blind Trial." *Arthritis and Rheumatism*. Jan.–Feb. 1973.

Gerner, H., D. A. Gorelick, D. H. Catlin, and C. H. Li. "Behavioral Effects of Beta-endorphin in Depression and Schizophrenia." *Endorphins and Opiate Antagonists in Psychiatric Research, Clinical Implications*. New York: Plenum Press, 1982.

Gold, Mark S., et al. "Epidemiology of Benzodiazepine Use and Dependence." *Psychiatric Annals* Vol. 25 No. 3, March, 1995, pp. 146–148.

Goldberg, I. "Tyrosine in Depression." *Lancet.* August 1980.

Goodheart, Robert S. and Maurice E. Shils. *Modern Nutrition in Health and Disease.* Philadelphia: Lea & Febiger, 1980, pp. 1220–1221.

Glenmullen, Joseph, M.D. *Prozac Backlash.* New York, NY: Simon & Schuster, 2000.

Grant, Larry A. "Amino Acids in Action." *Let's Live.* August, 1983, p. 63.

Greenstein, J. F. and M. Winitz. *Chemistry of the Amino Acids.* New York: Wiley Press, 1961.

Growden, A., Wurtman and Wurtman, eds. "Neurotransmitter Precursors in the Diet." *Nutrition and the Brain.* New York: Raven Press, 1979, pp. 117-181.

Hochman, Joel, A.V. Anderson, and Forest Tennant. "Antidepressants in Pain Treatment." *Practical Pain Management.* Jan./Feb. 2003, p. 12–14.

Hanson, H.C. "Treatment of chronic pain with antiepileptic drugs: a new era." *Southern Medical Journal.* July 1999, Vol. 92, No. 7, pp. 642–649.

Harper, Harold A. *Review of Physiological Chemistry.* Los Altos, California: Lange Medical Publications, 1969, p. 29.

Hart, Carol. *Secrets of Serotonin.* St. Martin Press, NY, 1996.

Heller, B. "Pharmacological and Clinical Effects of D-phenylalanine in Depression and Parkinson's Disease." *Modern Pharmacology-Toxicology.* 1985.

Hendler, Sheldon Saul and David Rorvik (ed). *PDR for Nutritional Supplements.* Montvale, NJ: Medical Economics Company. 2001.

Hoehn-Saric, R., et al. "Cerebral blood flow in obsessive-compulsive patients with major depression: effect of treatment with sertraline or desipramine on treatment responders and non-responders. *Psychiatry Research.* 2001. Vol. 108, pp. 89–100.

Hudson, J.I. and H.G. Pope. "Affective spectrum disorder: does antidepressant response identify a family of disorders with a common pathophysiology?" *American Journal of Psychiatry.* 1990. Vol. 147, pp. 552–564.

"Important Safety Information for Olanzapine." Eli Lilly Co. zyprexa.com, pp. 1–3.

Kagan, C., R. Griffith, and A. Norins. *Dermatologica*. Vol. 156. (1978).

Khaleeluddin, K. and W. Philpott. "Data Sheet." Philpott Medical Center, Oklahoma City, Oklahoma, 1980.

King, Robert B. "Pain and Tryptophan," *Journal Neurosurgery*. Vol. 53, July 1980, pp. 48-50.

Kotulak, Ronald. *Inside the Brain*. Kansas City: Andrews and McMeel, 1996.

Krawiec, Jeanne V. and Joanne M. Pohl. "Smoking Cessation and Nicotine Replacement Therapy. A Guide for Primary Car Providers." *American Journal for Nurse Practitioners*. Vol. 2. No. 1., January, 1998, pp. 15–33.

Lader, Malcolm. *Introductions to Psychopharmacology*. Kalamazoo, MI: The Upjohn Co., 1983, pp. 99-100.

Leibovitz, Brian. *Carnitine, The Vitamin BT Phenomenon*. New York: Dell Books, 1984, pp. 1318-1329.

LeDoux, Joseph, *The Emotional Brain,* New York, NY: Touchstone, 1996.

Leuchter, A. and R. Jaoin. "Addressing both the emotional and physical symptoms: beyond serotonin, two are better than one in treating depression. Program and abstracts of the 15th Annual *U.S. Psychiatric Congress*. October 28–31, 2002. Las Vegas, NV. Symposium 26-0.

"Lilly Announces FDA notification of Class Labeling for Atypical Antipsychotics Regarding Hyperglycemia and Diabetes." Eli Lilly and Company Press Release, Sept. 17, 2003.

Lynch, M.E. Antidepressants as analgesics: a review of randomized controlled trials." *Journal of Psychiatry Neuroscience*. 2001, Vol. 26, pp. 30–36.

Magni, G. "The use of antidepressants in the treatment of chronic pain. A review of the current evidence. *Drugs*. 1991, Vol. 42, pp. 730–748.

Mattia, C., et al. "New antidepressants in the treatment of neuropathic pain. A review." *Minerva Anesthesiology*. March 2002, Vol. 68 No. 3, pp. 105–114.

Maurer, I., H.P. Volz, and H. Sauer. "Gabapentin leads to remission of somatoform pain disorder with major depression." *Pharmacopsychiatry*. November 1999, Vol. 32 No. 6, pp. 255–257.

Maxmen, Jerrold S. and Nicholas G. Ward. *Psychotropic Drugs Fast Facts.* 2nd Ed. New York: W.W. Norton & Company, 1995.

Meister, A. *Biochemistry of the Amino Acids.* New York: Academic Press, 1975.

McQuay, H.J., et al. "A systematic review of antidepressants in neuropathic pain." *Pain.* Vol. 68, pp. 217–227.

Milam, James R. and Katherine Kethcam. *Under the Influence.* New York: Bantam Books, 1983), pp. 31, 37–38.

Miller, Norman S., et al. "Benzodiazepines: the Dissociation of Addiction." From Pharmacological Dependence/ Withdrawal." *Psychiatric Annuals* Vol. 25 No. 3, March, 1995, pp. 149–152.

Mills, Kirk C., M.D. "Serotonin Syndrome." *American Family Physician.* October 1995. p. 1475.

Miller, Norman S. "Liability and Efficacy From Long-Term Use of Benzodiazepines: Documentation and Interpretation." *Psychiatric Annals* Vol. 25 No. 3, March, 1995, pp. 166–173.

Moore, Thomas J. *Prescription for Disaster.* New York: Simon & Schuster, 1998.

Nardini, M., et al. "Treatment of depression with l-5-hydroxy-tryptophan combined with chlorimipramine: A double blind study. *Journal Clinical Pharmacology Research.* Vol. 2, 1983, pp. 239–250.

New Frontiers in Pain Control: Alternatives to Drugs and Surgery (Pacific Palisades, CA: Center for Intergral Medicine, 1978), p. 20.

Newbold, H. L. *Mega-Nutrients for Your Nerves.* New York: Peter Wyden Publishing, 1975.

National Institute of Drug Abuse (NIDA), US Department of Health.

Norden, Michael J. *Beyond Prozac. New* York, New York: HarperCollins Publisher, Inc., 1995

Nurse Practitioners' Prescribing Reference, Winter 2003, Volume 10, Number 4.

Omoigui, Sota. *The Pain Drugs Handbook.* St. Louis: Mosby, 1995.

"Patients using SSRIs may relapse if taken off too soon." *Psychopharmacology Update.* Vol. 9, No. 10, October 1998, pp. 1, 5–6.

Pauling, Linus. *Orthomolecular Psychiatry.* San Francisco: Freeman and Co., 1973.

Pearson, D., and R. Shaffer. *Nutritional Consultants.* November-December, 1980), p. 12.

Pearson, Durk and Sandy Shaw. *Alcohol.* Huntington Beach, California: International Institute of Natural Health Sciences, Inc., 1981, p. 20.

Pert, Candace B. "Letter to the Editor." *Time Magazine.* October 20, 1997, p. 80.

Pert, Candace B. *Molecules of Emotion*, New York, NY: Scribner, 1997.

Pfeiffer, Carl C. *Mental and Elemental Nutrients.* New Canaan, Connecticut: Keats Publishing Co., Inc., 1975, pp. 382-383.

Pfeiffer, Carl C., Ph.D., M.D., *Nutrition and Mental Illness*, Rochester, VT: 1987.

Phelps, Janice and Alan E. Nourse. *The Hidden Addiction and How to Get Free.* Boston: Little, Brown and Co., 1986, pp. 35–41, 79–85.

Physicians' Desk Reference. Montvale, NJ: Medical Economics Company, Inc., 56th Ed., 2002.

Pickens, Roy W. and Leonard L. Heston, eds. *Psychiatric Factors in Drug Abuse.* New York: Grune & Stratton, 1979, pp. 1–238.

Pickup, Dixon, Lowe, and Wright. "Serum Histidine in Rheumatoid Arthritis: Changes Induced by Antirheumatic Drug Therapy." *The Journal of Rheumatology.* Vol. 17, No. 1, 1980.

Pray, D.R. (ed.) "Pharmacologic Management of Depression: Length of Treatment, Treatment of the Elderly, and Selective Serotonin Reuptake Inhibitors." *Psychiatric Times, Special Report*, August 1993,.

Psychiatric Annals Vol. 25, No. 3, March 1995.

Psychopharmacology Update. Providence, RI: Manisses Communications Group, Inc., 1996.

Psychopharmacology Update. "News Update." Providence, RI: Manisses Communications Group, Inc., May, 1998, p. 5.

Rapp, Doris J. *Allergies and Your Family.* Buffalo: Practical Allergy Research Foundation, 2nd edition, 1990.

Ricketts, Max, with Edward Bien. *The Great Anxiety Escape.* La Mesa, CA: Matulungin Publishing, 1990.

RN Magazine's NDR-91. New York: Delmar Publishers, Inc., 1991.

Roe, Daphne A. *Drug-Induced Nutritional Deficiencies.* Westport, Connecticut: Avi Publishing Co., 1978, pp. 200–201, 204–208.

Rogers, Sherry. "Magnesium." Total Health & Wellness Letter. May-June 1995.

Rogers, Sherry A. *Pain Free in Six Weeks.* Sarasota, FL: Sand Key Co., Inc., 2001.

Rose, W. C., D. E. Leach, J. J. Coon, and G. F. Lamberg. "The Amino Acid Requirements of Man. The Phenylalanine Requirement." *The Journal of Biological Chemistry.* Vol. 213, 1955.

Rosenfeld, Isadore. "Heads Up, Migraine Sufferers." *Parade.* January 5, 2003, p. 19.

Rubin, Rita. "Prescription painkiller habit is easy to miss." *USA Today.* November 18, 2003, p. 7D.

Rudin, D.O., Felix, C. *The Omega-3 Phenomenon.* New York, NY: Rawson Associates, 1987.

Ruoff, G.E. "Depression in the patient with chronic pain." *Journal of Family Practice.* 1996, Vol. 43 (6 Suppl): S25–33; Discussion S34.

Russell, I.J. "New developments in the management of fibromyalgia syndrome." Program and abstracts of the *American College of Rheumatology 2002 Annual Meeting.* October 25–29, 2002, New Orleans, LA.

Sabelli, H. and A. D. Mosnaim. "Phenylethlamine Hypothesis of Affective Behavior." *American Journal of Psychiatry.* Vol. 131, 1974.

Sahley, Billie J., and Katherine M. Birkner. *Breaking Your Prescribed Addiction.* San Antonio, TX: Pain & Stress Publications, 1998.

Sahley, Billie J., and Katherine M. Birkner. *Heal With Amino Acids and Nutrients.* San Antonio, TX: Pain & Stress Publications, 2001.

Sahley, Billie J., Ph.D. *Theanine, the Relaxation Amino Acid.* San Antonio, TX: Pain & Stress Publications, 2004.

Sahley, Billie J. *The Anxiety Epidemic.* San Antonio, Texas: Pain & Stress Publications, 2002.

Saifer, Phyllis and Merla Zellerbach. *Detox.* New York: Ballantine Books, 1984, pp. 100, 101–105, 113, 135–137.

Salzman, Bernard. *The Handbook of Psychiatric Drugs.* New York: Henry Holt and Company, 1991.

Schatzberg, Alan F., and Charles B. Nemeroff. *The American Psychiatric Press Textbook of Psychopharmacology.* Washington, D.C.: American Psychiatric Press, Inc., 1995.

Schmidt, Michael A. *Smart Fats: How Dietary Fats and Oils Affect Mental, Physical and Emotional Intelligence.* Berkeley, CA: Frog, Ltd., 1997.

Seelig, Mildred S. and Andrea Rosanoff. *The Magnesium Factor.* New York, NY: Penguin Group, 2003.

"Seroquel Package Insert." AstraZeneca Pharmaceuticals, Jan. 04.

Shader, Richard I., ed. *Manual of Psychiatric Therapeutics.* Boston: Little, Brown, and Co., 1984, pp. 213, 273, 289.

Shader, Richard I., *Brain.* New York: Raven Press, 1979.

Sherman, C. "Longterm side effects surface with SSRIs: insomnia, weight gain, sexual dysfunction emerge as problems affecting compliance." *Clinical Psychiatry News*, 1998, pp. 4–5.

Shive, W., et al. "Glutamine in Treatment of Peptic Ulcer," *Texas State Journal of Medicine.* Vol. 53 (1957).

Slagle, Priscilla. *The Way Up From Down.* New York: St. Martin's Press, 1987, pp. 113, 142–145, 149, 241–247.

Smith, Bernard H. and Antonio Rosich-Pla. "The Biochemistry of Mental Illness." *Psychosomatics.* April, 1979, p. 282.

Smith, Lendon. *Feed Yourself Right.* New York: Dell Publishing Co., Inc., 1983, pp. 33, 108, 112.

Sodhi, Virender, M.D., N.D., *Ashwagandha for Rejuvenation*, New Editions Health World, 2000.

Solvay Pharmaceuticals. "Luvox, A Selective Serotonin Reuptake Inhibitor." Information booklet, 1995.

Spatz, H., B. Heller, M. Nachon, and E. Fischer. "Effects of D-phenylalanine on Clinical Picture and Phenylethylaminuria in Depression." *Biological Psychiatry.* Vol. 10, No. 2, 1975.

Stahl, S.M. "Basic psychopharmacology of antidepressants: part 1: antidepressants have seven distinct mechanisms of action. *Journal of Clinical Psychiatry.* Vol. 59, 1998. (Suppl 4), pp. 5–14.

Stein, et al. "Memory Enhancement by Central Administration of Norepinephrine." *Brain Research.* Vol. 84, 1975, pp. 329–335.

Shute, Wilfrid E. *Health Preserver.* Emmaus, PA: Rodale Press, 1977.

Stubbs, C.D. "The structure and function of docosahexaenoic acid in membranes." In Sinclair, A, Gibson, R, eds., *Essential Fatty Acids and Eicosanoids.* Champaign, IL: American Oil Chemists' Society, 1992, p. 116.

Tennant, Forest, Laura Herman, Leah Silliman, and Jeffrey Reinking. "Identifying Pain-Drug Abusers and Addicts." *Practical Pain Management.* Nov./Dec. 2002, pp. 21–26.

Trickett, Shirley. *Coming Off Tranquilizers.* New York: Thorson Publishing Group, 1986.

Thomas, Clayton L., ed. *Taber's Cyclopedic Medical Dictionary.* Philadelphia: PA. Davis Company, 1993.

Tornatore, Frank L., et al. *Reactions to Psychotropic Medications.* New York: Plenum Medical Book Co., 1987.

Van der Kolk, B., Dreyfuss, D., Michaels, M., et al. "Fluoxetine in post-traumatic stress disorder." *Journal of Clinical Psychiatry*, Vol. 55. No. 12,1994, pp. 517–522.

Verma, S. and R.M. Gallagher. "The psychopharmacolic treatment of depression and anxiety in the context of chronic pain." *Current Pain Headache Report.* Vol. 6, 2002 , pp. 30–39.

White, A., et al. *Principles of Biochemistry.* New York: McGraw-Hill, 1978, pp. 1120, 1241–1264.

Wolfe, Sidney M., M.D. and Rose-Ellen Hope, R.Ph. *Worst Pills Best Pills II.* Washington, DC: Public Citizen Health Research Group. 1993.

Wright, Jonathan V., M.D. "Lithium, Protect and Renew Your Brain, Parts I and II" *Townsend Letter for Doctors and Patients*, February/March, 2004, pp. 78–81.

Woodman, Sue. "Pill of 1,001 Uses." *My Generation.* September-October 2001.

Index

Other Resources

Books . . .

The Antidepressant Fact Book (Peter Breggin, M.D.)

Inside the Brain, Revolutionary Discoveries of How the Mind Works (Ronald Kotulak)

Over Dose, The Case Against the Drug Companies (Jay. S. Cohen, M.D.)

Prozac Backlash (Josepth Glenmullen, M.D.)

Toxic Psychiatry (Peter Breggin, M.D.)

Your Drug May Be Your Problem (Peter Breggin, M.D.)

Pain Free in 6 Weeks (Sherry A. Rogers, M.D.)

Tape . . .

Amino Acids & How They Effect Brain Function
Audio Tape (Billie J. Sahley, Ph.D.)

Presented at the Academy of Functional Medicine Conference
March 22, 2003

Topics include using amino acids with anxiety, depression, chronic pain, grief, panic, fear, stress, etc.

Dr. Sahley discusses the importance of neurotransmitters from amino acids and their effect on brain functions. She explains how to use amino acids including dosages. You must put back in the brain what belongs there in specific amounts to correct a chemical imbalance.

Serotonin is the master controller. GABA is the anxiety amino acid. L-T is the relaxation amino acid. Amino acids are the keys to enhanced mind, mood, memory, and behavior.

Dr. Sahley gives an educational and informative hour packed with information you will use daily.

**Books and Tapes are available at 1-800-669-2256 OR
go to http://www.painstresscenter.com**

Dr. Billie Sahley is available for lectures. Call the Pain & Stress Mgmt. Clinic for more information at 210-614-7246.

Other Books From
Pain & Stress Publications

To Order Call 1-800-669-2256 or
go to http://www.painstresscenter.com

About The Authors

Billie J. Sahley, Ph.D., is Executive Director of the Pain & Stress Center in San Antonio. She is a Board Certified Medical Psychotherapist & Psychodiagnostician, Behavior Therapist, Orthomolecular Therapist, and a Certified Nutritional Consultant. She is a Diplomate in the American Academy of Pain Management. Dr. Sahley is a graduate of the University of Texas, Clayton University School of Behavioral Medicine, and U.C.L.A. School of Integral Medicine. Additionally, she has studied advanced nutritional biochemistry through Jeffrey Bland, Ph.D., Director of HealthComm. She is a member of the Huxley Foundation/Academy of Orthomolecular Medicine, American Academy of Environmental Medicine, Academy of Psychosomatic Medicine, North American Nutrition and Preventive Medicine Association, and American Counseling Association. In addition, she holds memberships in the Sports Medicine Foundation, American Association of Hypnotherapists, and American Mental Health Counselors Association. She also sits on the Scientific and Medical Advisory Board for Inter-Cal Corporation.

Dr. Sahley wrote: *The Anxiety Epidemic; GABA, The Anxiety Amino Acid; Post Trauma and Chronic Emotional Fatigue; Malic Acid and Magnesium For Fibromyalgia and Chronic Pain Syndrome; The Melatonin Report; Is Ritalin Necessary? The Ritalin Report; Stop A.D.D. Naturally; Theanine, The Relaxation Amino Acid;* and has recorded numerous audiocassette tapes. She coauthored *Heal With Amino Acids*.

In addition, Dr. Sahley holds three U.S. patents for: SAF, Calms Kids (SAF For Kids), and Anxiety Control 24. Dr. Sahley devotes the majority of her time to research, writing, and development of natural products to address brain deficiencies.

Kathy Birkner is a C.R.N.A., Pain Therapist at the Pain & Stress Center in San Antonio. She is a Registered Nurse, Certified Registered Nurse Anesthetist, Advanced Nurse Practitioner, Orthomolecular Therapist, and a Certified Nutritional Consultant. She is a Diplomate in the American Academy of Pain Management. She attended Brackenridge Hospital School of Nursing, University of Texas at Austin, Southwest Missouri School of Anesthesia, Southwest Missouri State University, and Clayton University. She holds degrees in nursing, nutrition, and behavior therapy. Dr. Birkner has done graduate studies through the Center for Integral Medicine and U.C.L.A. Medical School, under the direction of Dr. David Bresler. Additionally, she has studied advanced nutritional biochemistry through Jeffrey Bland, Ph.D., Director of HealthComm. She is a member of the American Association of Nurse Anesthetists, Texas Association of Nurse Anesthetists, American Association of Pain Management, American College of Osteopathic Pain Management and Sclerotherapy. She is author of *Breaking Your Sugar Habit Cookbook* and the book, *Heal with Amino Acids*.